Burning Mouth Syndrome

Tests, Causes and Treatment Options

John Smith MA

© 2014 John Smith MA

All Rights Reserved worldwide under the Berne Convention. May not be copied or distributed without prior written permission by the publisher.

ISBN 978-1497363212

Contents

Contents

One: What is Burning Mouth Syndrome (BMS)?............ 5
Two: Causes and Risks... 7
    Diabetes mellitus..12
    Candidiasis 42
    Nutrition disorder 51
    References..54
Three: Symptoms and signs 71
Four: Meeting the doctor for BMS..............................75
Five: Tests and diagnosis of BMS................................81
Six: Treatment 85
Seven: Lifestyle Changes...89
Glossary of Medical Terms 93
Appendix A: Internet Resources / Further Reading . 111

One: What is Burning Mouth Syndrome (BMS)?

Burning mouth syndrome – also known as burning tongue or orodynia -- is a condition where you feel a burning sensation in your mouth. This pain can affect many parts of your mouth like the lips, tongue and gums. It may cause pain in the roof of your mouth or its walls. In some cases, it may even affect your throat.

This condition is a result of a neuropathic disorder. This means that your nerves start to malfunction. They don't send the correct information to the brain or don't process brain's signals correctly. The result is that you have a constant burning sensation in your mouth.

There are no definite causes known which result in burning mouth syndrome. It can be a result of some other underlying mouth disease or a physical medical disorder. However, with proper care and medication, this condition can be controlled.

The condition is much more prevalent among women than men. In fact, women have a seven times greater risk of suffering from it than men. Also, burning mouth syndrome mostly occurs in middle age people. It occurs less often in young people. About one million people in the U.S. alone are affected by this condition.

Burning mouth syndrome is also given a number of other names such as scalded mouth syndrome, glossodynia, stomatodynia, burning tongue syndrome and burning lips syndrome.

Two: Causes and Risks

Although no clear causes are known for this condition, doctors suggest that it may be a result of other diseases. These include:

Diabetes mellitus. It has not been proven that diabetes mellitus causes burning mouth syndrome. But doctors think that there's a high chance that a relationship exists between diabetes mellitus and burning mouth syndrome (BMS). So if you are diabetic and also suffer from BMS, your doctor will suggest you to take very good care of your diabetes. Lipoic acid is helpful for diabetics and some doctors think that it may be helpful in treating BMS.

Xerostomia, a condition which causes dry mouth due to low saliva production. It is a common condition in older people. It starts when the salivary glands start to malfunction and do not produce normal amounts of saliva. This make you feel as if your mouth is very dry. Dry mouth is sometimes an outcome of using certain medications. About 400 drugs are said to cause this condition, e.g., anticholinergic and sympathomimetics.

Other **oral infections** such as a tongue yeast infection (thrush, or candidiasis).

Menopause. This results in an imbalance of hormones in the body of women and can result in burning mouth syndrome. Most women suffer from burning mouth syndrome immediately after menopause.

AIDS. If you have AIDS, the immune system of the body becomes very weak and you become vulnerable to a number of diseases. Due to this weak immune system, certain infections may also occur in your body which can give birth to burning mouth syndrome.

Psychological factors such as **depression, anxiety** and heightened worry about something. This can be a result of a sudden accident that can cause trauma. Such trauma can lead to a number of abnormalities in the body, including BMS.

Nutritional deficiency, especially a deficiency of vitamin B2 (riboflavin). A lack of iron, vitamin B1 (thiamin), zinc, Vitamin B6 (pyridoxine) and vitamin B12 (cobalamin) may also cause burning mouth syndrome. This is usually treated by taking in a regular dose of supplements. For example, if you are suffering from iron deficiency and that has caused your BMS, your doctor will suggest you to take iron supplements.

Dentures are an artificial replacement for the damaged teeth. These dentures may result in a reaction from the muscles and tissues of the mouth, causing pain and burning mouth syndrome. Sometimes, if an inexperienced dentist has operated on your teeth and hasn't done it properly, it may lead to infections. Such infections may cause a burning sensation in the mouth and lead to BMS.

Allergies. If you are allergic to a certain food which causes pain in your tooth or which your mouth-tissues are sensitive to, taking that food may cause burning mouth syndrome. It may be a little difficult to find out exactly what kind of foods you are allergic to. You can discover it by carefully noticing your diet and its effect on your body. When you experience the symptoms of burning mouth syndrome, you should immediately note what you have eaten recently. This will help your doctor diagnose if there is any allergy you are suffering from and whether that allergy has caused BMS.

Some **medications** can also cause this condition. For example, angiotensin-converting enzyme (ACE) inhibitors, which are used to treat high blood pressure (hypertension), can result in this condition.

Increased taste sensation. This is a common symptom of BMS and that's why doctors think that it may cause the condition in many people. However, that claim is not proven. Increased taste sensation means that you start tasting everything more clearly and intensely than normal. Something which is normally not so spicy may seem very spicy to you due to this condition. This happens because the density of taste buds on your tongue increases.

Trigeminal Nerve Neuropathy, a condition which results in periods of intense pain in the face.

Gastroesophageal reflux disease (GERD), a condition in which stomach acid rises through the esophagus – the path leading from the mouth to the stomach.

Usually, your doctor won't be able to determine what caused your mouth burning syndrome. In such a case, it is called primary burning mouth syndrome. But if your condition is a result of another underlying disease, such as those mentioned above, then it is called secondary burning mouth syndrome. Secondary BMS is easy to treat as the doctor is able to identify the cause. Its treatment is also not very long-term.

Normally, this condition starts all of a sudden without any warning. But there are some things that can increase the chances of you getting this condition. These factors are listed here:

An infection of your throat or lungs.

An event that makes you suffer emotionally. For example, if you survive an accident, it may lead you to trauma and anxiety .And that can increase the risks of you getting burning mouth syndrome.

Being careless towards diet and eating foods that you are allergic to. If you are not careful enough to avoid such foods to which your mouth or body are sensitive, it may result in this condition.

Incorrect dental procedures by a poor dentist. If you had your teeth incorrectly operated on by a dentist, it can lead to infections and teeth problems. It can also result in a reaction by your mouth tissues and muscles. All this can lead to burning mouth syndrome.

There is no known cure that directly treats burning mouth syndrome. This is because so far, doctors have not been able to define what causes this condition. In about one-third of the cases, it is a result of some other disease. In other cases, the cause is unknown. So, all the known treatments for burning mouth syndrome are aimed at the other underlying conditions which cause it. For example, if a hormonal imbalance is causing burning mouth syndrome in your case, your doctor will treat you so that the hormonal imbalance is cured. This automatically leads to a cure of burning mouth syndrome. But if the cause is unknown, the doctor has no idea what is the right medication for you. In such a case, the doctor only takes a guess and suggests a medication according to that guess. You may not feel any better by using that medicine and then your doctor will change the medication. And so, he will keep suggesting medications and changing them if they have no affect on your condition until you hit on the right medication. Because of this, the treatment of primary type of BMS can take a very long time. It may even take years for your BMS to completely go away.

Diabetes mellitus

Diabetes mellitus, often simply referred to as **diabetes**, is a group of metabolic diseases in which a person has high blood sugar, either because the body does not produce enough insulin, or because cells do not respond to the insulin that is produced. This high blood sugar produces the classical symptoms of polyuria(frequent urination), polydipsia(increased thirst) and polyphagia(increased hunger).

There are three main types of diabetes:

Type 1 diabetes: results from the body's failure to produce insulin, and presently requires the person to inject insulin. (Also referred to as *insulin-dependent* diabetes mellitus, *IDDM* for short, and *juvenile* diabetes.)

Type 2 diabetes: results from insulin resistance, a condition in which cells fail to use insulin properly, sometimes combined with an absolute insulin deficiency. (Formerly referred to as *non-insulin-dependent* diabetes mellitus, *NIDDM* for short, and *adult-onset* diabetes.)

Gestational diabetes: is when pregnant women, who have never had diabetes before, have a high blood glucose level during pregnancy. It may precede development of type 2 DM.

Other forms of diabetes mellitus include congenital diabetes, which is due to genetic defects of insulin secretion, cystic fibrosis-related diabetes, steroid diabetes induced by high doses of glucocorticoids, and several forms of monogenic diabetes.

All forms of diabetes have been treatable since insulin became available in 1921, and type 2 diabetes may be controlled with medications. Both type 1 and 2 are chronic conditions that usually cannot be cured. Pancreas transplantshave been tried with limited success in type 1 DM; gastric bypass surgery has been successful in many with morbid obesity and type 2 DM. Gestational diabetes usually resolves after delivery. Diabetes without proper treatments can cause many complications. Acute complications include hypoglycemia,diabetic ketoacidosis, or nonketotic hyperosmolar coma. Serious long-term complications include cardiovascular disease, chronic renal failure, retinal damage. Adequate treatment of diabetes is thus important, as well as blood pressure control and lifestyle factors such as smoking cessation and maintaining a healthy body weight.

As of 2000 at least 171 million people worldwide have diabetes, or 2.8% of the population.[2] Type 2 diabetes is by far the most common, affecting 90 to 95% of the U.S. diabetes population.[3]

Classification

Most cases of diabetes mellitus fall into three broad categories: type 1, type 2, and gestational diabetes. A few other types are described. The term *diabetes*, without qualification, usually refers to diabetes *mellitus*. The rare disease diabetes insipidus has similar symptoms as diabetes mellitus, but without disturbances in the sugar metabolism (insipidus meaning "without taste" in Latin).

Comparison of type 1 and 2 diabetes		
Feature	**Type 1 diabetes**	**Type 2 diabetes**
Onset	Sudden[4]	Gradual[4]
Age at onset	Any age (mostly young)[4]	Mostly in adults
Body habitus	Thin[4] or normal[5]	Often obese[4]
Ketoacidosis	Common[4]	Rare[4]
Autoantibodies	Usually present[4]	Absent[4]
Endogenous insulin	Low or absent[4]	Normal, decreased or increased[4]
Concordance in identical twins	50%[4]	90%[4]
Prevalence	Less prevalent	More prevalent - 90 to 95% of U.S. diabetics[3]

The term "type 1 diabetes" has replaced several former terms, including childhood-onset diabetes, juvenile diabetes, and insulin-dependent diabetes mellitus (IDDM). Likewise, the term "type 2 diabetes" has replaced several former terms, including adult-onset diabetes, obesity-related diabetes, and non-insulin-dependent diabetes mellitus (NIDDM). Beyond these two types, there is no agreed-upon standard nomenclature. Various sources have defined "type 3 diabetes" as: gestational diabetes,[6] insulin-resistant type 1 diabetes (or "double diabetes"), type 2 diabetes which has progressed to require injected insulin, and latent autoimmune diabetes of adults (or LADA or "type 1.5" diabetes).[7]

Type 1 diabetes

Type 1 diabetes mellitus is characterized by loss of the insulin-producing beta cells of the islets of Langerhans in the pancreas leading to insulin deficiency. This type of diabetes can be further classified as immune-mediated or idiopathic. The majority of type 1 diabetes is of the immune-mediated nature, where beta cell loss is a T-cell mediated autoimmune attack.[8] There is no known preventive measure against type 1 diabetes, which causes approximately 10% of diabetes mellitus cases in North America and Europe. Most affected people are otherwise healthy and of a healthy weight when onset occurs. Sensitivity and responsiveness to insulin are usually normal, especially in the early stages. Type 1 diabetes can affect children or adults but was traditionally termed "juvenile diabetes" because it represents a majority of the diabetes cases in children.

Brittle diabetes, also known as unstable diabetes or labile diabetes, refers to a type of insulin-dependent diabetes characterized by dramatic and recurrent swings in glucose levels, often occurring for no apparent reason.[9] The result can be irregular and unpredictable hyperglycemias, frequently with ketosis, and sometimes serious hypoglycemias. Brittle diabetes occurs no more frequently than in 1% to 2% of diabetics.[10]

Type 2 diabetes

Type 2 diabetes mellitus is characterized by insulin resistance which may be combined with relatively reduced insulin secretion. The defective responsiveness of body tissues to insulin is believed to involve the insulin receptor. However, the specific defects are not known. Diabetes mellitus due to a known defect are classified separately. Type 2 diabetes is the most common type.

In the early stage of type 2 diabetes, the predominant abnormality is reduced insulin sensitivity. At this stage hyperglycemia can be reversed by a variety of measures and medications that improve insulin sensitivity or reduce glucose production by the liver.

Gestational diabetes

Gestational diabetes mellitus (GDM) resembles type 2 diabetes in several respects, involving a combination of relatively inadequate insulin secretion and responsiveness. It occurs in about 2%–5% of all pregnancies and may improve or disappear after delivery. Gestational diabetes is fully treatable but requires careful medical supervision throughout the pregnancy. About 20%–50% of affected women develop type 2 diabetes later in life.

Even though it may be transient, untreated gestational diabetes can damage the health of the fetus or mother. Risks to the baby include macrosomia (high birth weight), congenital cardiac and central nervous system anomalies, and skeletal muscle malformations. Increased fetal insulin may inhibit fetal surfactant production and cause respiratory distress syndrome. Hyperbilirubinemia may result from red blood cell destruction. In severe cases, perinatal death may occur, most commonly as a result of poor placental perfusion due to vascular impairment. Labor induction may be indicated with decreased placental function. A cesarean section may be performed if there is marked fetal distress or an increased risk of injury associated with macrosomia, such as shoulder dystocia.

A 2008 study completed in the U.S. found that the

number of American women entering pregnancy with preexisting diabetes is increasing. In fact the rate of diabetes in expectant mothers has more than doubled in the past 6 years.[11] This is particularly problematic as diabetes raises the risk of complications during pregnancy, as well as increasing the potential that the children of diabetic mothers will also become diabetic in the future.

Other types

Pre-diabetes indicates a condition that occurs when a person's blood glucose levels are higher than normal but not high enough for a diagnosis of type 2 diabetes. Many people destined to develop type 2 diabetes spend many years in a state of pre-diabetes which has been termed "America's largest healthcare epidemic."[12]:10–11

Latent autoimmune diabetes of adults is a condition in which Type 1 diabetes develops in adults. Adults with LADA are frequently initially misdiagnosed as having Type 2 diabetes, based on age rather than etiology.

Some cases of diabetes are caused by the body's tissue receptors not responding to insulin (even when insulin levels are normal, which is what separates it from type 2 diabetes); this form is very uncommon. Genetic mutations (autosomal or mitochondrial) can lead to defects in beta cell function. Abnormal insulin action may also have been genetically determined in some cases. Any disease that causes extensive damage to the pancreas may lead to diabetes (for example, chronic pancreatitis and cystic fibrosis). Diseases associated with excessive secretion of insulin-antagonistic hormones can cause diabetes (which is typically resolved once the hormone excess is removed). Many drugs impair insulin secretion and some toxins damage pancreatic beta cells. The ICD-10 (1992) diagnostic entity, *malnutrition-related diabetes mellitus* (MRDM or MMDM, ICD-10 code E12), was deprecated by the World Health Organization when the current taxonomy was introduced in 1999.[13]

Signs and symptoms

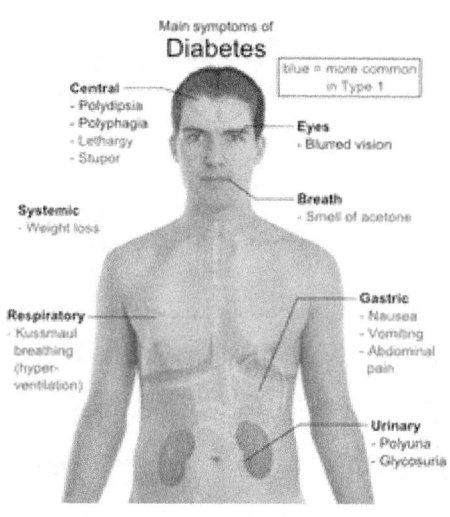

Overview of the most significant symptoms of diabetes.

Hyperglycemia and osmosis

The classical symptoms of diabetes are polyuria (frequent urination), polydipsia (increased thirst) and polyphagia (increased hunger).[114] Symptoms may develop rapidly (weeks or months) in type 1 diabetes while in type 2 diabetes they usually develop much more slowly and may be subtle or absent.

Prolonged high blood glucose causes glucose absorption, which leads to changes in the shape of the lenses of the eyes, resulting in vision changes; sustained sensible glucose control usually returns the lens to its original shape. Blurred vision is a common complaint leading to a diabetes diagnosis; type 1 should always be suspected in cases of rapid vision change, whereas with type 2 change is generally more gradual, but should still be suspected

Diabetic emergencies

People (usually with type 1 diabetes) may also present with diabetic ketoacidosis, a state of metabolic dysregulation characterized by the smell of acetone; a rapid, deep breathing known as Kussmaul breathing; nausea; vomiting and abdominal pain; and altered states of consciousness.

A rarer but equally severe possibility is hyperosmolar nonketotic state, which is more common in type 2 diabetes and is mainly the result of dehydration. Often, the patient has been drinking extreme amounts of sugar-containing drinks, leading to a vicious circle in regard to the water loss.

Complications

All forms of diabetes increase the risk of long-term complications. These typically develop after many years (10–20), but may be the first symptom in those who have otherwise not received a diagnosis before that time. The major long-term complications relate to damage to blood vessels.

Diabetes doubles the risk of cardiovascular disease.[15] The main "macrovascular" diseases (related to atherosclerosis of larger arteries) are ischemic heart disease (angina and myocardial infarction), stroke and peripheral vascular disease.

Diabetes also causes "microvascular" complications—damage to the small blood vessels.[16] Diabetic retinopathy, which affects blood vessel formation in the retina of the eye, can lead to visual symptoms, reduced vision, and potentially blindness. Diabetic nephropathy, the impact of diabetes on the kidneys, can lead to scarring changes in the kidney tissue, loss of small or progressively larger amounts of protein in the urine, and eventually chronic kidney disease requiring dialysis. Diabetic neuropathy is the impact of diabetes on the nervous system, most commonly causing numbness, tingling and pain in the feet and also increasing the risk of skin damage due to altered sensation. Together with vascular disease in the legs, neuropathy contributes to the risk of diabetes-related foot problems (such as diabetic foot ulcers) that can be difficult to treat and occasionally require amputation.

Other problems

A number of skin rashes can occur in diabetes that are collectively known as diabetic dermadromes.

Causes

The cause of diabetes depends on the type.

Type 1 diabetes is partly inherited and then triggered by certain infections, with some evidence pointing at Coxsackie B4 virus. There is a genetic element in individual susceptibility to some of these triggers which has been traced to particular HLA genotypes (i.e., the genetic "self" identifiers relied upon by the immune system). However, even in those who have inherited the susceptibility, type 1 diabetes mellitus seems to require an environmental trigger.

Type 2 diabetes is due primarily to lifestyle factors and genetics.[17]

Following is a comprehensive list of other causes of diabetes:[18]

Genetic defects of β-cell Function

Maturity onset diabetes of the young (MODY)

Endocrinopathies

Growth hormone excess (acromegaly)

Cushing syndrome

Mitochondrial DNA mutations
Genetic defects in insulin processing or insulin action
Defects in proinsulin conversion
Insulin gene mutations
Insulin receptor mutations
Exocrine Pancreatic Defects
Chronic pancreatitis
Pancreatectomy
Pancreatic neoplasia
Cystic fibrosis
Hemochromatosis
Fibrocalculous pancreatopathy

Hyperthyroidism
Pheochromocytoma
Glucagonoma
Infections
Cytomegalovirus infection
Coxsackievirus B
Drugs
Glucocorticoids
Thyroid hormone
β-adrenergic agonists

Pathophysiology

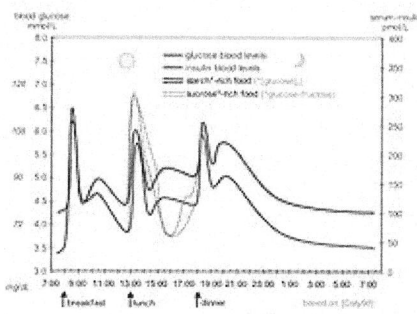

The fluctuation of blood sugar (red) and the sugar-lowering hormone insulin (blue) in humans during the course of a day with three meals. One of the effects of a sugar-rich vs a starch-rich meal is highlighted.

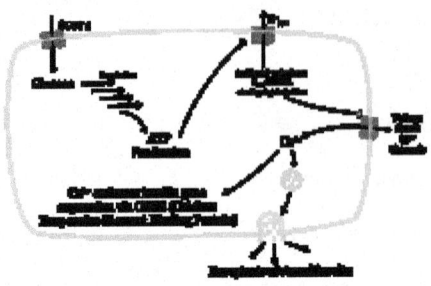

Mechanism of insulin release in normal pancreatic beta cells. Insulin production is more or less constant within the beta cells. Its release is triggered by food, chiefly food containing absorbable glucose.

Insulin is the principal hormone that regulates uptake of glucose from the blood into most cells (primarily muscle and fat cells, but not central nervous system cells). Therefore deficiency of insulin or the insensitivity of its receptors plays a central role in all forms of diabetes mellitus.

Humans are capable of digesting some carbohydrates, in particular those most common in food; starch, and some disaccharides such as sucrose, are converted within a few hours to simpler forms most notably the monosaccharide glucose, the principal carbohydrate energy source used by the body. The rest are passed on for processing by gut flora largely in the colon. Insulin is released into the blood by beta cells (β-cells), found in the Islets of Langerhans in the pancreas, in response to rising levels of blood glucose, typically after eating. Insulin is used by about two-thirds of the body's cells to absorb glucose from the blood for use as fuel, for conversion to other needed molecules, or for storage.

Insulin is also the principal control signal for conversion of glucose to glycogen for internal storage in liver and muscle cells. Lowered glucose levels result both in the reduced release of insulin from the beta cells and in the reverse conversion of glycogen to glucose when glucose levels fall. This is mainly controlled by the hormone glucagon which acts in the opposite manner to insulin. Glucose thus forcibly produced from internal liver cell stores (as glycogen) re-enters the bloodstream; muscle cells lack the necessary export mechanism. Normally liver cells do this when the level of insulin is low (which normally correlates with low levels of blood glucose).

Higher insulin levels increase some anabolic ("building up") processes such as cell growth and duplication, protein synthesis, and fat storage. Insulin (or its lack) is the principal signal in converting many of the bidirectional processes of metabolism from a catabolic to an anabolic direction, and vice versa. In particular, a low insulin level is the trigger for entering or leaving ketosis (the fat burning metabolic phase).

If the amount of insulin available is insufficient, if cells respond poorly to the effects of insulin (insulin insensitivity or resistance), or if the insulin itself is defective, then glucose will not have its usual effect so that glucose will not be absorbed properly by those body cells that require it nor will it be stored appropriately in the liver and muscles. The net effect is persistent high levels of blood glucose, poor protein synthesis, and other metabolic derangements, such as acidosis.

When the glucose concentration in the blood is raised beyond its renal threshold (about 10 mmol/L, although this may be altered in certain conditions, such as pregnancy), reabsorption of glucose in the proximal renal tubuli is incomplete, and part of the glucose remains in the urine (glycosuria). This increases the osmotic pressure of the urine and inhibits reabsorption of water by the kidney, resulting in increased urine production (polyuria) and increased fluid loss. Lost blood volume will be replaced osmotically from water held in body cells and other body compartments, causing dehydration and increased thirst.

Diagnosis

Glucose tolerance test

2006 WHO Diabetes criteria[19]

Condition	2 hour glucose mmol/l (mg/dl)	Fasting glucose mmol/l(mg/dl)
Normal	<7.8 (<140)	<6.1 (<110)
Impaired fasting glycaemia	<7.8 (<140)	≥ 6.1(≥110) & <7.0(<126)
Impaired glucose tolerance	≥7.8 (≥140)	<7.0 (<126)
Diabetes mellitus	≥11.1 (≥200)	≥7.0 (≥126)

Diabetes mellitus is characterized by recurrent or persistent hyperglycemia, and is diagnosed by demonstrating any one of the following:[13]

Fasting plasma glucose level ≥ 7.0 mmol/L (126 mg/dL).

Plasma glucose ≥ 11.1 mmol/L (200 mg/dL) two hours after a 75 g oral glucose load as in a glucose tolerance test.

Symptoms of hyperglycemia and casual plasma glucose ≥ 11.1 mmol/L (200 mg/dL).

Glycated hemoglobin (Hb A1C) ≥ 6.5%.[20]

A positive result, in the absence of unequivocal hyperglycemia, should be confirmed by a repeat of any of the above-listed methods on a different day. It is preferable to measure a fasting glucose level because of the ease of measurement and the considerable time commitment of formal glucose tolerance testing, which takes two hours to complete and offers no prognostic advantage over the fasting test.[21] According to the current definition, two fasting glucose measurements above 126 mg/dL (7.0 mmol/L) is considered diagnostic for diabetes mellitus.

People with fasting glucose levels from 100 to 125 mg/dL (5.6 to 6.9 mmol/L) are considered to have impaired fasting glucose. Patients with plasma glucose at or above 140 mg/dL (7.8 mmol/L), but not over 200 mg/dL (11.1 mmol/L), two hours after a 75 g oral glucose load are considered to have impaired glucose tolerance. Of these two pre-diabetic states, the latter in particular is a major risk factor for progression to full-blown diabetes mellitus as well as cardiovascular disease.[22]

Glycated hemoglobin is better than fasting glucose for determining risks of cardiovascular disease and death from any cause.[23]

Management

Diabetes mellitus is a chronic disease which cannot be

cured except in very specific situations. Management concentrates on keeping blood sugar levels as close to normal ("euglycemia") as possible, without causing hypoglycemia. This can usually be accomplished with diet, exercise, and use of appropriate medications (insulin in the case of type 1 diabetes, oral medications as well as possibly insulin in type 2 diabetes).

Patient education, understanding, and participation is vital since the complications of diabetes are far less common and less severe in people who have well-managed blood sugar levels.[24][25] The goal of treatment is an HbA1C level of 6.5%, but should not be lower than that, and may be set higher.[26] Attention is also paid to other health problems that may accelerate the deleterious effects of diabetes. These include smoking, elevated cholesterol levels, obesity, high blood pressure, and lack of regular exercise.[26]

Lifestyle

There are roles for patient education, dietetic support, sensible exercise, with the goal of keeping both short-term and long-term blood glucose levels within acceptable bounds. In addition, given the associated higher risks of cardiovascular disease, lifestyle modifications are recommended to control blood pressure.[27]

Medications

Oral medications

Metformin is generally recommended as a first line treatment for type 2 diabetes as there is good evidence that it decreases mortality.[28] Routine use of aspirin however has not been found to improve outcomes in uncomplicated diabetes.[29]

Insulin

Type 1 diabetes is typically treated with a combinations of regular and NPH insulin, or synthetic insulin analogs. When insulin is used in type 2 diabetes, a long-acting formulation is usually added initially, while continuing oral medications.[28] Doses of insulin are then increased to effect.[28]

Support

In countries using a general practitioner system, such as the United Kingdom, care may take place mainly outside hospitals, with hospital-based specialist care used only in case of complications, difficult blood sugar control, or research projects. In other circumstances, general practitioners and specialists share care of a patient in a team approach. Optometrists,podiatrists/chiropodists, dietitians, physiotherapists, nursing specialists (e.g., DSNs (Diabetic Specialist Nurse)), nurse practitioners, or certified diabetes educators, may jointly provide multidisciplinary expertise.

Epidemiology

[33]

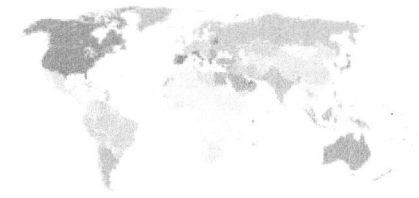

In 2000, according to the World Health Organization, at least 171 million people worldwide suffer from diabetes, or 2.8% of the population.[2] Its incidence is increasing rapidly, and it is estimated that by 2030, this number will almost double.[2] Diabetes mellitus occurs throughout the world, but is more common (especially type 2) in the more developed countries. The greatest increase in prevalence is, however, expected to occur in Asia and Africa, where most patients will probably be found by 2030.[2] The increase in incidence of diabetes in developing countries follows the trend of urbanization and lifestyle changes, perhaps most importantly a "Western-style" diet. This has suggested an environmental (i.e., dietary) effect, but there is little understanding of the mechanism(s) at present, though there is much speculation, some of it most compellingly presented.[2]

Prevalence in the United States

For at least 20 years, diabetes rates in North America have been increasing substantially. In 2010 nearly 26 million people have diabetes in the United States alone, from those 7 million people remain undiagnosed. Another 57 million people are estimated to have pre-diabetes.[30]

The Centers for Disease Control has termed the change an epidemic.[31] The National Diabetes Information Clearinghouse estimates that diabetes costs $132 billion in the United States alone every year. About 5%–10% of diabetes cases in North America are type 1, with the rest being type 2. The fraction of type 1 in other parts of the world differs. Most of this difference is not currently understood. The American Diabetes Association cite the 2003 assessment of the National Center for Chronic Disease Prevention and Health Promotion (Centers for Disease Control and Prevention) that 1 in 3 Americans born after 2000 will develop diabetes in their lifetime.[32][33]

According to the American Diabetes Association, approximately 18.3% (8.6 million) of Americans age 60 and older have diabetes.[34] Diabetes mellitus prevalence increases with age, and the numbers of older persons with diabetes are expected to grow as the elderly population increases in number. The National Health and Nutrition Examination Survey (NHANES III) demonstrated that, in the population over 65 years old, 18% to 20% have diabetes, with 40% having either diabetes or its precursor form of impaired glucose tolerance.[35]

Prevalence in Australia

Indigenous populations in first world countries have a

higher prevalence and increasing incidence of diabetes than their corresponding non-indigenous populations. In Australia the age-standardised prevalence of self-reported diabetes in Indigenous Australians is almost 4 times that of non-indigenous Australians.[36] Preventative community health programs such as Sugar Man (diabetes education) are showing some success in tackling this problem.

Etymology

The word "diabetes"

(🔊 /ˌdaɪ.ə.ˈbiː.tiːz/ or /ˌdaɪ.ə.ˈbiː.tɨs/) comes from Latin *diabētēs*, which in turn comes from Ancient Greek διαβήτης (*diabētēs*) which literally means "a passer through; a siphon."[37] Ancient Greek physician Aretaeus of Cappadocia (fl. 1st century CE) used that word, with the intended meaning "excessive discharge of urine," as the name for the disease.[38][39] Ultimately, the word comes from Greek διαβαίνειν (*diabainein*), meaning "to pass through,"[37] which is composed of δια- (*dia-*), meaning "through" and βαίνειν (*bainein*), meaning "to go".[38] The word "diabetes" is first recorded in English, in the form *diabete*, in a medical text written around 1425.

The word "*mellitus*"

(/mɨ.ˈlaɪ.təs/ or /ˈmɛ.lɨ.təs/) comes from the classical Latin word *mellītus*, meaning "mellite"[40] (i.e.

sweetened with honey;[40] honey-sweet[41]). The Latin word comes from *mell-*, which comes from *mel*, meaning "honey;[40][41] sweetness;[41] pleasant thing,[41]" and the suffix -*itus*,[40] whose meaning is the same as that of the English suffix "-ite."[42] It was Thomas Willis who in 1675 added "mellitus" to the word "diabetes" as a designation for the disease, when he noticed that the urine of a diabetic had a sweet taste (glycosuria).[39] This sweet taste had been noticed in urine by the ancient Greeks, Chinese, Egyptians, Indians, and Persians.

History

Diabetes is one of the oldest known diseases.[39] An Egyptian manuscript from c. 1550 BCE mentions the phrase "the passing of too much urine."[39] The great Indian physician Sushruta (fl. 6th century BCE)[39] identified the disease and classified it as *Medhumeha*.[43] He further identified it with obesity and sedentary lifestyle, advising exercises to help "cure" it.[43] The ancient Indians tested for diabetes by observing whether ants were attracted to a person's urine, and called the ailment "sweet urine disease" (Madhumeha).

Concerning the sweetness of urine, it is to be noted that the Chinese, Japanese and Korean words for diabetes are based on the same ideographs (糖尿病) which mean "sugar urine disease". It was in 1776 that Matthew Dobson confirmed that the sweet taste comes from an excess of a kind of sugar in the urine and blood.[44]

The first complete clinical description of diabetes was given by the Ancient Greek physician Aretaeus of Cappadocia (fl. 1st century CE), who noted the excessive amount of urine which passed through the kidneys and gave the disease the name "diabetes."[39]

Diabetes mellitus appears to have been a death sentence in the ancient era. Hippocrates makes no mention of it, which may indicate that he felt the disease was incurable. Aretaeus did attempt to treat it but could not give a good prognosis; he commented that "life (with diabetes) is short, disgusting and painful."[45]

In medieval Persia, Avicenna (980–1037) provided a detailed account on diabetes mellitus in *The Canon of Medicine*, "describing the abnormal appetite and the collapse of sexual functions," and he documented the sweet taste of diabetic urine. Like Aretaeus before him, Avicenna recognized a primary and secondary diabetes. He also described diabetic gangrene, and treated diabetes using a mixture of lupine, trigonella (fenugreek), and zedoary seed, which produces a considerable reduction in the excretion of sugar, a treatment which is still prescribed in modern times. Avicenna also "described diabetes insipidus very precisely for the first time", though it was later Johann Peter Frank (1745–1821) who first differentiated between diabetes mellitus and diabetes insipidus.[46]

Although diabetes has been recognized since antiquity, and treatments of various efficacy have been known in various regions since the Middle Ages, and in legend for much longer, pathogenesis of diabetes has only been understood experimentally since about 1900.[47] The discovery of a role for the pancreas in diabetes is generally ascribed to Joseph von Mering and Oskar Minkowski, who in 1889 found that dogs whose pancreas was removed developed all the signs and symptoms of diabetes and died shortly afterwards.[48] In 1910, Sir Edward Albert Sharpey-Schafer suggested that people with diabetes were deficient in a single chemical that was normally produced by the pancreas—he proposed calling this substance *insulin*, from the Latin *insula*, meaning island, in reference to the insulin-producing islets of Langerhans in the pancreas.

The endocrine role of the pancreas in metabolism, and indeed the existence of insulin, was not further clarified until 1921, when Sir Frederick Grant Banting and Charles Herbert Best repeated the work of Von Mering and Minkowski, and went further to demonstrate they could reverse induced diabetes in dogs by giving them an extract from the pancreatic islets of Langerhans of healthy dogs.[49] Banting, Best, and colleagues (especially the chemist Collip) went on to purify the hormone insulin from bovine pancreases at the University of Toronto. This led to the availability of an effective treatment—insulin injections—and the first patient was treated in 1922. For this, Banting and laboratory director MacLeod received the Nobel Prize in Physiology or Medicine in 1923; both shared their Prize money with others in the team who were not recognized, in particular Best and Collip. Banting and Best made the patent available without charge and did not attempt to control commercial production. Insulin production and therapy rapidly spread around the world, largely as a result of this decision. Banting is honored by World Diabetes Day which is held on his birthday, November 14.

The distinction between what is now known as type 1 diabetes and type 2 diabetes was first clearly made by Sir Harold Percival (Harry) Himsworth, and published in January 1936.[50]

Despite the availability of treatment, diabetes has remained a major cause of death. For instance, statistics reveal that the cause-specific mortality rate during 1927 amounted to about 47.7 per 100,000 population in Malta.[51]

Other landmark discoveries include:[47]

Identification of the first of the sulfonylureas in 1942

Reintroduction of the use of biguanides for Type 2 diabetes in the late 1950s. The initial phenformin was withdrawn worldwide (in the U.S. in 1977) due to its potential for sometimes fatal lactic acidosis and metformin was first marketed in France in 1979, but not until 1994 in the US.

The determination of the amino acid sequence of insulin (by Sir Frederick Sanger, for which he received a Nobel Prize)

The radioimmunoassay for insulin, as discovered by Rosalyn Yalow and Solomon Berson (gaining Yalow the 1977 Nobel Prize in Physiology or Medicine)[52]

The three-dimensional structure of insulin (PDB 2INS)

Dr Gerald Reaven's identification of the constellation of symptoms now called metabolic syndrome in 1988

Demonstration that intensive glycemic control in type 1 diabetes reduces chronic side effects more as glucose levels approach 'normal' in a large longitudinal study,[53] and also in type 2 diabetics in other large studies

Identification of the first thiazolidinedione as an effective insulin sensitizer during the 1990s

In 1980, U.S. biotech company Genentech developed biosynthetic human insulin. The insulin was isolated from genetically altered bacteria (the bacteria contain the human gene for synthesizing synthetic human insulin), which produce large quantities of insulin. The purified insulin is distributed to pharmacies for use by diabetes patients.

Initially, this development was not regarded by the medical profession as a clinically meaningful development. However, by 1996, the advent of insulin analogues which had vastly improved absorption, distribution, metabolism, and excretion (ADME) characteristics which were clinically meaningful based on this early biotechnology development.

Society and culture

The 1990 "St. Vincent Declaration"[54][55] was the result of international efforts to improve the care accorded to those with diabetes. Doing so is important both in terms of quality of life and life expectancy but also economically— expenses due to diabetes have been shown to be a major drain on health-and productivity-related resources for healthcare systems and governments.

Several countries established more and less successful national diabetes programmes to improve treatment of the disease.[56]

A study shows that diabetic patients with neuropathic symptoms such as numbness or tingling in feet or hands are twice as likely to be unemployed as those without the symptoms.[57]

In other animals

In animals, diabetes is most commonly encountered in dogs and cats. Middle-aged animals are most commonly affected. Male dogs are twice as likely to be affected as females, while according to some sources male cats are also more prone than females. In both species, all breeds may be affected, but some small dog breeds are particularly likely to develop diabetes, such as Miniature Poodles.[58] The symptoms may relate to fluid loss and polyuria, but the course may also be insidious. Diabetic animals are more prone to infections. The long-term complications recognised in humans are much rarer in animals. The principles of treatment (weight loss, oral antidiabetics, subcutaneous insulin) and management of emergencies (e.g. ketoacidosis) are similar to those in humans.[58]

Candidiasis

Candidiasis or **thrush** is a fungal infection (mycosis) of any of the *Candida* species (all yeasts), of which *Candida albicans* is the most common.[1][2] Also commonly referred to as a **yeast infection**, candidiasis is also technically known as **candidosis, moniliasis,** and **oidiomycosis**.[3]:308

Candidiasis encompasses infections that range from superficial, such as oral thrush and vaginitis, to systemic and potentially life-threatening diseases. *Candida* infections of the latter category are also referred to as candidemia and are usually confined to severely immunocompromised persons, such as cancer, transplant, and AIDS patients as well as non-trauma emergency surgery patients.[4]

Superficial infections of skin and mucosal membranes by *Candida* causing local inflammation and discomfort are common in many human populations.[2][5][6] While clearly attributable to the presence of the opportunistic pathogens of the genus *Candida*, candidiasis describes a number of different disease syndromes that often differ in their causes and outcomes.[2][5]

Classification

Candidiasis may be divided into the following types:[3]:308–311

Oral candidiasis (Thrush)

Perlèche (Angular cheilitis)

Candidal vulvovaginitis (vaginal yeast infection)

Candidal intertrigo

Diaper candidiasis

Congenital cutaneous candidiasis

Perianal candidiasis

Candidal paronychia

Erosio interdigitalis blastomycetica

Chronic mucocutaneous candidiasis

Systemic candidiasis

Candidid

Antibiotic candidiasis (Iatrogenic candidiasis)

Signs and symptoms

Most candidial infections are treatable and result in minimal complications such as redness, itching and discomfort, though complication may be severe or fatal if left untreated in certain populations.

In immunocompetent persons, candidiasis is usually a very localized infection of the skin or mucosal membranes, including the oral cavity (thrush), the pharynx or esophagus, the gastrointestinal tract, the urinary bladder, or the genitalia (vagina, penis).[1]

Candidiasis is a very common cause of vaginal irritation, or vaginitis, and can also occur on the male genitals. In immunocompromised patients, *Candida* infections can affect the esophagus with the potential of becoming systemic, causing a much more serious condition, a fungemia called candidemia.[5][6]

Thrush is commonly seen in infants. It is not considered abnormal in infants unless it lasts longer than a couple of weeks.[7]

Children, mostly between the ages of three and nine years of age, can be affected by chronic mouth yeast infections, normally seen around the mouth as white patches. However, this is not a common condition.

Symptoms of candidiasis may vary depending on the area affected. Infection of the vagina or vulva may cause severe itching, burning, soreness, irritation, and a whitish or whitish-gray cottage cheese-like discharge, often with a curd-like appearance. These symptoms are also present in the more common bacterial vaginosis.[8] In a 2002 study published in the *Journal of Obstetrics and Gynecology*, only 33 percent of women who were self-treating for a yeast infection actually had a yeast infection, while most had either bacterial vaginosis or a mixed-type infection.[9] Symptoms of infection of the male genitalia include red patchy sores near the head of the penis or on the foreskin, severe itching, or a burning sensation. Candidiasis of the penis can also have a white discharge, although uncommon.

Causes

Candida yeasts are commonly present in humans, and their growth is normally limited by the human immune system and by other microorganisms, such as bacteria occupying the same locations (niches) in the human body.[10]

C. albicans was isolated from the vaginas of 19% of apparently healthy women, i.e., those that experienced few or no symptoms of infection. External use of detergents or douches or internal disturbances (hormonal or physiological) can perturb the normal vaginal flora, consisting of lactic acid bacteria, such as lactobacilli, and result in an overgrowth of *Candida* cells causing symptoms of infection, such as local inflammation.[11] Pregnancy and the use of oral contraceptives have been reported as risk factors,[12] while the roles of engaging in vaginal sex immediately and without cleansing after anal sex and using lubricants containing glycerin remain controversial.[1] Diabetes mellitus and the use of anti-bacterial antibiotics are also linked to an increased incidence of yeast infections.[12] Diet high in carbohydrates has been found to affect rates of oral candidiases,[13] and hormone replacement therapy and infertility treatments may also be predisposing factors.[14] Wearing wet swimwear for long periods of time is also believed to be a risk factor.[2]

A weakened or undeveloped immune system or metabolic illnesses such as diabetes are significant predisposing factors of candidiasis.[15] Diseases or conditions linked to candidiasis include HIV/AIDS, mononucleosis, cancertreatments, steroids, stress, and nutrient deficiency. Almost 15% of people with weakened immune systems develop a systemic illness caused by *Candida* species.[16] In extreme cases, these superficial infections of the skin or mucous membranes may enter into the bloodstream and cause systemic *Candida* infections.

In penile candidiasis, the causes include sexual intercourse with an infected individual, low immunity, antibiotics, and diabetes. Male genital yeast infection is less common, and incidence of infection is only a fraction of that in women; however, yeast infection on the penis from direct contact via sexual intercourse with an infected partner is not uncommon.[17]

Candida species are frequently part of the human body's normal oral and intestinal flora. Treatment with antibiotics can lead to eliminating the yeast's natural competitors for resources, and increase the severity of the condition. Higher prevalence of colonization of *C. albicans* was reported in young individuals with tongue piercing, in comparison to non-tongue-pierced matched individuals.[18] In the western hemisphere approximately 75% of females are affected at some time in their life.

Diagnosis

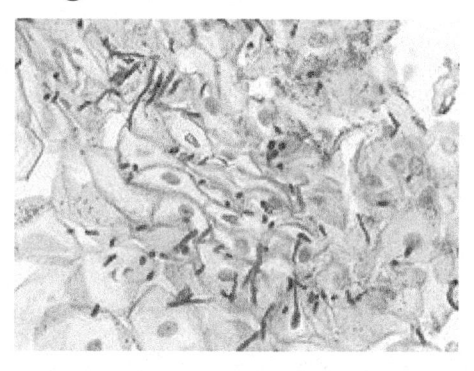

Micrograph of esophageal candidiasis.Biopsy specimen; PAS stain.

Diagnosis of a yeast infection is done either via microscopic examination or culturing.

For identification by light microscopy, a scraping or swab of the affected area is placed on amicroscope slide. A single drop of 10% potassium hydroxide (KOH) solution is then added to the specimen. The KOH dissolves the skin cells but leaves the *Candida*cells intact, permitting visualization of pseudohyphae and budding yeast cells typical of many *Candida* species.

For the culturing method, a sterile swab is rubbed on the infected skin surface. The swab is then streaked on a culture medium. The culture is incubated at 37 °C for several days, to allow development of yeast or bacterial colonies. The characteristics (such as morphology and colour) of the colonies may allow initial diagnosis of the organism that is causing disease symptoms. [19]

Treatment

In clinical settings, candidiasis is commonly treated with antimycotics—theantifungal drugs commonly used to treat candidiasis are topical clotrimazole, topical nystatin, fluconazole, and topical ketoconazole.

For example, a one-time dose of fluconazole (150-mg tablet taken orally) has been reported as being 90% effective in treating a vaginal yeast infection.[20]This dose is only effective for vaginal yeast infections, and other types of yeast infections may require different dosing. In severe infections amphotericin B,caspofungin, or voriconazole may be used. Local treatment may include vaginal suppositories or medicated douches. Gentian violet can be used for breastfeeding thrush, but when used in large quantities it can cause mouth and throat ulcerations in nursing babies, and has been linked to mouth cancer in humans and to cancer in the digestive tract of other animals.[21]

Chlorhexidine gluconate oral rinse is not recommended to treat candidiasis[22] but is effective as prophylaxis;[23] chlorine dioxide rinse was found to have similar in vitro effectiveness against *candida*.[24]

C. albicans can develop resistance to antimycotic drugs.[25] Recurring infections may be treatable with other anti-fungal drugs, but resistance to these alternative agents may also develop.

History

The genus *Candida* and species *C. albicans* was described by botanist Christine Marie Berkhout in her doctoral thesis at the University of Utrecht in 1923. Over the years, the classification of the genera and species has evolved. Obsolete names for this genus include *Mycotorula* and *Torulopsis*. The species has also been known in the past as *Monilia albicans* and *Oidium albicans*. The current classification is *nomen conservandum*, which means the name is authorized for use by the International Botanical Congress (IBC).[26]

The genus *Candida* includes about 150 different species, however, only a few are known to cause human infections: *C. albicans* is the most significantpathogenic species. Other *Candida* species pathogenic in humans include *C. tropicalis*, *C. glabrata*, *C. krusei*, *C. parapsilosis*, *C. dubliniensis*, and *C. lusitaniae*.

Society and culture

Some alternative medicine proponents postulate a widespread occurrence of systemic candidiasis (or candida hypersensitivity syndrome, yeast allergy, or gastrointestinal candida overgrowth). The view was most widely promoted in a book published by Dr. William Crook,[27] which hypothesized that a variety of common symptoms such as fatigue, PMS, sexual dysfunction, asthma, psoriasis, digestive and urinary problems, multiple sclerosis, and muscle pain, could be caused by subclinical infections of *Candida albicans*.[27] Crook suggested a variety of remedies to treat these symptoms, ranging from dietary modification, prescription antifungals, to colonic irrigation. With the exception of the few dietary studies in the urinary tract infection section, conventional medicine has not used most of these alternatives, since there is limited scientific evidence to prove either their effectiveness, or that subclinical systemic candidiasis is a viable diagnosis.[28][29][30][31]

Nutrition disorder

Nutritional diseases are diseases in humans that are directly or indirectly caused by a lack of essential nutrients in the diet. Nutritional diseases are commonly associated with chronic malnutrition. Additionally, conditions such as obesity from overeating can also cause, or contribute to, serious health problems. Excessive intake of some nutrients can cause acute poisoning.

Overnutrition

Metabolic

Obesity is caused by consuming too many calories compared to the amount of exercise the body is performing, causing a distorted energy balance. It can lead to diseases such as cardiovascular disease and diabetes. Obesity is a condition in which the natural energy reserve, stored in the fatty tissue of humans and other mammals, is increased to a point where it is associated with certain health conditions or increased mortality.

The low-cost food that is generally affordable to the poor in affluent nations is low in nutritional value and high in fats, sugars and additives. In rich countries, therefore, obesity is oftentimes a sign of poverty and malnutrition while in poorer countries obesity is more associated with wealth and good nutrition. Other non-nutritional causes for unhealthy obesity included: sleep deprivation, stress, lack of exercise, and heredity.

Acute overeating can also be a symptom of an eating disorder.

Goitrogenic foods can cause goitres by interfering with iodine uptake.

Vitamins and micronutrients

Vitamin poisoning is the condition of overly high storage levels of vitamins, which can lead to toxic symptoms. The medical names of the different conditions are derived from the vitamin involved: an excess of vitamin A, for example, is called "hypervitaminosis A".

Iron overload disorders are diseases caused by the overaccumulation of iron in the body. Organs commonly affected are the liver, heart and endocrine glands in the mouth.

Deficiencies

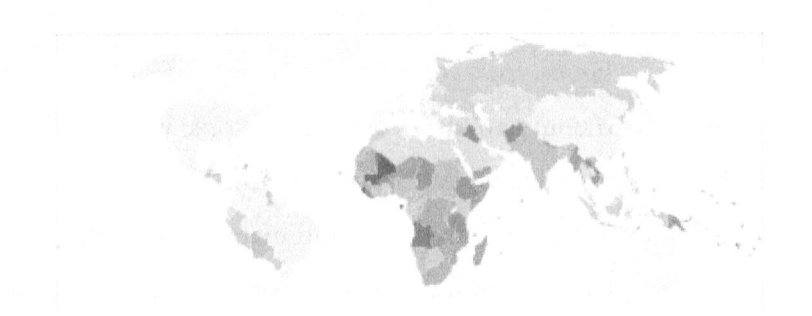

Proteins/fats/carbohydrates

Protein-energy malnutrition

Kwashiorkor

Marasmus

Mental retardation[2]

Dietary vitamins and minerals

Calcium

Osteoporosis

Rickets

Tetany

Iodine deficiency

Goiter

Selenium deficiency

Keshan disease

Iron deficiency

Iron deficiency anemia

Zinc

Growth retardation

Thiamine (Vitamin B_1)

Beriberi

Niacin (Vitamin B_3)

Pellagra

Vitamin C

Scurvy

Vitamin D

Osteoporosis

Rickets

Complex disorders

In some cases, eating too much of one thing can induce an apparent deficiency of something else. A common example occurs when livestock eat locoweed: locoweed contains a toxin that inhibits enzymes, simulating a deficiency of the enzymes.

Foot notes

^ "Mortality and Burden of Disease Estimates for WHO Member States in 2002" (xls).*World Health Organization.* 2002.

^ "Malnutrition Is Cheating Its Survivors, and Africa's Future"article in the New York Times by Michael Wines, December 28, 2006

From Wikipedia, the free encyclopedia: http://en.wikipedia.org/wiki/Nutritional_deficiencies

References

References -- Candidiasis

[a,b] Walsh TJ, Dixon DM (1996)."Deep Mycoses". In Baron S *et al.* eds.. *Baron's Medical Microbiology* (4th ed.). Univ of Texas Medical Branch. ISBN 0-9631172-1-1.

[a b c d] MedlinePlus Encyclopedia *Vaginal yeast infection*

[a b] James, William D.; Berger, Timothy G.; et al. (2006). *Andrews' Diseases of the Skin: clinical Dermatology*. Saunders Elsevier.ISBN 0-7216-2921-0.

http://en.wikipedia.org/wiki/Candidiasis - cite_ref-3 Kourkoumpetis T, Manolakaki D, Velmahos G, *et al.* (2010)."Candida infection and colonization among non-trauma emergency surgery patients".*Virulence* **1** (5): 359–66.doi:10.4161/viru.1.5.12795.PMID 21178471.

[a b c] Fidel PL (2002). "Immunity to Candida". *Oral Dis.* **8**: 69–75.doi:10.1034/j.1601-0825.2002.00015.x.PMID 12164664.

[a b] Pappas PG (2006). "Invasive candidiasis". *Infect. Dis. Clin. North Am.* **20** (3): 485–506.doi:10.1016/j.idc.2006.07.004.PMID 16984866.

http://en.wikipedia.org/wiki/Candidiasis - cite_ref-6 "Thrush". 2011. Retrieved 2011-04-08.

http://en.wikipedia.org/wiki/Candidiasis - cite_ref-7 Terri Warren, RN (2010). "Is It a Yeast Infection?". Retrieved 2011-02-23.

http://en.wikipedia.org/wiki/Candidiasis - cite_ref-8 Ferris DG; Nyirjesy P; Sobel JD; Soper D; Pavletic A; Litaker MS (March 2002). "Over-the-counter antifungal drug misuse associated with patient-diagnosed vulvovaginal candidiasis". *Obstetrics and Gynecology* **99** (3): 419–

425.doi:10.1016/S0029-7844(01)01759-8.PMID 11864668.

http://en.wikipedia.org/wiki/Candidiasis - cite_ref-9 Mulley, A. G.; Goroll, A. H. (2006).*Primary Care Medicine: office evaluation and management of the adult patient.* Philadelphia: Wolters Kluwer Health. pp. 802–3.ISBN 0-7817-7456-X. Retrieved 2008-11-23.

http://en.wikipedia.org/wiki/Candidiasis - cite_ref-10 Mårdh P A, Novikova N, Stukalova E (October 2003)."Colonisation of extragenital sites by Candida in women with recurrent vulvovaginal candidosis". *BJOG* **110** (10): 934–7. doi:10.1111/j.1471-0528.2003.01445.x.PMID 14550364.

[a,b] Schiefer HG (1997). "Mycoses of the urogenital tract".*Mycoses* **40** (Suppl 2): 33–6.doi:10.1111/j.1439-0507.1997.tb00561.x.PMID 9476502.

http://en.wikipedia.org/wiki/Candidiasis - cite_ref-Review2002_12-0 Akpan, A; Morgan, R (2002 Aug)."Oral candidiasis".*Postgraduate medical journal* **78**(922): 455–9.doi:10.1136/pmj.78.922.455.PMC 1742467.PMID 12185216.

http://en.wikipedia.org/wiki/Candidiasis - cite_ref-13 Nwokolo N C, Boag F C (May 2000). "Chronic vaginal candidiasis. Management in the postmenopausal patient". *Drugs Aging* **16** (5): 335–9.PMID 10917071.

http://en.wikipedia.org/wiki/Candidiasis - cite_ref-

Odds 14-0 Odds FC (1987). "Candida infections: an overview". *Crit. Rev. Microbiol.* **15** (1): 1–5.doi:10.3109/10408418709104444. PMID 3319417.

http://en.wikipedia.org/wiki/Candidiasis - cite_ref-15 Choo Z.W., Chakravarthi S., Wong S.F., Nagaraja H.S., Thanikachalam P.M., Mak J.W., Radhakrishnan A., Tay A. (2010)."A comparative histopathological study of systemic candidiasis in association with experimentally induced breast cancer".*Oncology Letters* **1** (1): 215–222.doi:10.3892/ol_00000039.ISSN 1792-1082.

http://en.wikipedia.org/wiki/Candidiasis - cite_ref-16 David LM, Walzman M, Rajamanoharan S (October 1997). "Genital colonisation and infection with candida in heterosexual and homosexual males". *Genitourin Med* **73** (5): 394–6. PMC 1195901.PMID 9534752.

http://en.wikipedia.org/wiki/Candidiasis - cite_ref-Candida_17-0 Zadik Yehuda, Burnstein Saar, Derazne Estella, Sandler Vadim, Ianculovici Clariel, Halperin Tamar (March 2010). "Colonization of Candida: prevalence among tongue-pierced and non-pierced immunocompetent adults". *Oral Dis* **16** (2): 172–5.doi:10.1111/j.1601-0825.2009.01618.x.PMID 19732353.

http://en.wikipedia.org/wiki/Candidiasis - cite_ref-18 Srikumar Chakravarthi, Nagaraja HS (2010). "A comprehensive review of the occurrence and management of systemic candidiasis as an opportunistic infection".*Microbiology Journal* **1** (2): 1–5.ISSN 2153-0696.

http://en.wikipedia.org/wiki/Candidiasis - cite_ref-Moosa_19-0 Moosa MY, Sobel JD, Elhalis H, Du W, Akins RA (2004)."Fungicidal Activity of Fluconazole against Candida albicans in a Synthetic Vagina-Simulative Medium". *Antimicrob. Agents Chemother.* **48** (1): 161–7.doi:10.1128/AAC.48.1.161-167.2004. PMC 310176.PMID 14693534.

http://en.wikipedia.org/wiki/Candidiasis - cite_ref-20 Craigmill A (December 1991)."Gentian Violet Policy Withdrawn". *Cooperative Extension University of California -- Environmental Toxicology Newsletter* **11** (5).

http://en.wikipedia.org/wiki/Candidiasis - cite_ref-21 "Chlorhexidine Gluconate". Drugs.Com. Retrieved Jan 8, 2011.

http://en.wikipedia.org/wiki/Candidiasis - cite_ref-22 Ferretti GA, Ash RC, Brown AT, Parr MD, Romond EH, Lillich TT (September 1988). "Control of oral mucositis and candidiasis in marrow transplantation: a prospective, double-blind trial of chlorhexidine digluconate oral rinse". *Bone Marrow Transplant.* **3**(5): 483–93. PMID 3056555.

http://en.wikipedia.org/wiki/Candidiasis - cite_ref-23 Uludamar A, Ozkan YK, Kadir T, Ceyhan I (2010). "In vivo efficacy of alkaline peroxide tablets and mouthwashes on

Candida albicans in patients with denture stomatitis". *J Appl Oral Sci* **18**(3): 291–6. doi:10.1590/S1678-77572010000300017.PMID 20857010.

http://en.wikipedia.org/wiki/Candidiasis - cite_ref-24 Cowen LE, Nantel A, Whiteway MS (July 2002). "Population genomics of drug resistance in Candida albicans". *Proc. Natl. Acad. Sci. U.S.A.* **99** (14): 9284–9.doi:10.1073/pnas.102291099.PMC 123132.PMID 12089321.

http://en.wikipedia.org/wiki/Candidiasis - cite_ref-25 *International Code of Botanical Nomenclature*. Königstein. 2000. ISBN 3-904144-22-7. Retrieved 2008-11-23.

[a,b] Crook, William G. (1986). *The yeast connection: a medical breakthrough*. New York: Vintage Books. ISBN 0394747003.

http://en.wikipedia.org/wiki/Candidiasis - cite_ref-27 Weil A (2002-10-25)."Concerned About Candidiasis?". Weil Lifestyle. Retrieved 2008-02-21.

http://en.wikipedia.org/wiki/Candidiasis - cite_ref-28 Barrett S (2005-10-08)."Dubious "Yeast Allergies"". QuackWatch. Retrieved 2008-02-21.

http://en.wikipedia.org/wiki/Candidiasis - cite_ref-29 Katherine Zeratsky. "Candida cleanse: Does it treat candidiasis?". Mayo Clinic. Retrieved 2009-08-09.

http://en.wikipedia.org/wiki/Candidiasis - cite_ref-

30 Blonz ER (December 1986). "Is there an epidemic of chronic candidiasis in our midst?"(PDF). *JAMA* **256** (22): 3138–9.doi:10.1001/jama.1986.03380220104032. PMID 3783850.

From Wikipedia the Free Encyclopedia: Candidiasis
http://en.wikipedia.org/wiki/Candidiasis

References -- Diabetes

http://en.wikipedia.org/wiki/Diabetes - cite_ref-0 "Diabetes Blue Circle Symbol". International Diabetes Federation. 17 March 2006.

[a][b][c][d][e] Wild S, Roglic G, Green A, Sicree R, King H (May 2004). "Global prevalence of diabetes: estimates for 2000 and projections for 2030". *Diabetes Care* **27** (5): 1047–53.doi:10.2337/diacare.27.5.1047.PMID 15111519.

[a][b] "Type 2 Diabetes Overview". Web MD.

[a][b][c][d][e][f][g][h][i][j][k][l][m] Elizabeth D Agabegi; Agabegi, Steven S. (2008). *Step-Up to Medicine (Step-Up Series)*. Hagerstwon, MD: Lippincott Williams & Wilkins.ISBN 0-7817-7153-6.

http://en.wikipedia.org/wiki/Diabetes - cite_ref-4 Lambert, P. (2002). "What is Type 1 Diabetes?". *Medicine* **30**: 1–5.doi:10.1383/medc.30.1.1.28264.

http://en.wikipedia.org/wiki/Diabetes - cite_ref-5 "Other "types" of diabetes".American Diabetes

Association. August 25, 2005.

http://en.wikipedia.org/wiki/Diabetes - cite_ref-6 "Diseases: Johns Hopkins Autoimmune Disease Research Center". Retrieved 2007-09-23.

http://en.wikipedia.org/wiki/Diabetes - cite_ref-Rother_7-0 Rother KI (April 2007). "Diabetes treatment—bridging the divide".*The New England Journal of Medicine* **356** (15): 1499–501.doi:10.1056/NEJMp078030.PMID 17429082.

http://en.wikipedia.org/wiki/Diabetes - cite_ref-8 "Diabetes Mellitus (DM): Diabetes Mellitus and Disorders of Carbohydrate Metabolism: Merck Manual Professional". Merck.com. Retrieved 2010-07-30.

http://en.wikipedia.org/wiki/Diabetes - cite_ref-pmid406527_9-0 Dorner M, Pinget M, Brogard JM (May 1977). "Essential labile diabetes" (in German). *MMW Munch Med Wochenschr* **119** (19): 671–4. PMID 406527.

http://en.wikipedia.org/wiki/Diabetes - cite_ref-10 Lawrence JM, Contreras R, Chen W, Sacks DA (May 2008). "Trends in the prevalence of preexisting diabetes and gestational diabetes mellitus among a racially/ethnically diverse population of pregnant women, 1999–2005". *Diabetes Care* **31**(5): 899–904. doi:10.2337/dc07-2345. PMID 18223030.

http://en.wikipedia.org/wiki/Diabetes - cite_ref-

11 Handelsman Yehuda, MD. "A Doctor's Diagnosis: Prediabetes".*Power of Prevention* **1** (2): 2009.

a b World Health OrganisationDepartment of Noncommunicable Disease Surveillance (1999)."Definition, Diagnosis and Classification of Diabetes Mellitus and its Complications" (PDF).

http://en.wikipedia.org/wiki/Diabetes - cite_ref-13 Cooke DW, Plotnick L (November 2008). "Type 1 diabetes mellitus in pediatrics".*Pediatr Rev* **29** (11): 374–84; quiz 385. doi:10.1542/pir.29-11-374.PMID 18977856.

http://en.wikipedia.org/wiki/Diabetes - cite_ref-14 "Diabetes mellitus, fasting blood glucose concentration, and risk of vascular disease: a collaborative meta-analysis of 102 prospective studies : The Lancet".

http://en.wikipedia.org/wiki/Diabetes - cite_ref-15 Boussageon R, Bejan-Angoulvant T, Saadatian-Elahi M,*et al.* (2011). "Effect of intensive glucose lowering treatment on all cause mortality, cardiovascular death, and microvascular events in type 2 diabetes: meta-analysis of randomised controlled trials".*BMJ* **343**: d4169.doi:10.1136/bmj.d4169.PMC 3144314.PMID 21791495.

http://en.wikipedia.org/wiki/Diabetes - cite_ref-Fat2009_16-0 Risérus U, Willett WC, Hu FB (January 2009). "Dietary fats and prevention of type 2 diabetes".*Progress in Lipid Research* **48** (1): 44–51.doi:10.1016/j.plipres.2008.10.002. PMC 2654180.PMID 19032965.

http://en.wikipedia.org/wiki/Diabetes - cite_ref-Robbins_17-0 Unless otherwise specified, reference is: Table 20-5 inMitchell, Richard Sheppard; Kumar, Vinay; Abbas, Abul K.; Fausto, Nelson. *Robbins Basic Pathology*. Philadelphia: Saunders. ISBN 1-4160-2973-7.8th edition.

http://en.wikipedia.org/wiki/Diabetes - cite_ref-who2006_18-0 "Definition and Diagnosis of Diabetes Mellitus and Intermediate Hyperglycemia"(pdf). *World Health Organization*. www.who.int. 2006. Retrieved 2011-02-20.

http://en.wikipedia.org/wiki/Diabetes - cite_ref-19 ""Diabetes Care" January 2010". *American Diabetes Association*. Retrieved 2010-01-29.

http://en.wikipedia.org/wiki/Diabetes - cite_ref-20 Saydah SH, Miret M, Sung J, Varas C, Gause D, Brancati FL (August 2001). "Postchallenge hyperglycemia and mortality in a national sample of U.S. adults".*Diabetes Care* **24** (8): 1397–402.doi:10.2337/diacare.24.8.1397.PMID 11473076.

http://en.wikipedia.org/wiki/Diabetes - cite_ref-21 Santaguida PL, Balion C, Hunt D, Morrison K, Gerstein H, Raina P, Booker L, Yazdi H. "Diagnosis, Prognosis, and Treatment of Impaired Glucose Tolerance and Impaired

Fasting Glucose". *Summary of Evidence Report/Technology Assessment, No. 128*. Agency for Healthcare Research and Quality. Retrieved 2008-07-20.

http://en.wikipedia.org/wiki/Diabetes - cite_ref-22 Selvin E, Steffes MW, Zhu H *et al*(2010). "Glycated hemoglobin, diabetes, and cardiovascular risk in nondiabetic adults". *N. Engl. J. Med.* **362** (9): 800–11.doi:10.1056/NEJMoa0908359.PMC 2872990.PMID 20200384.

http://en.wikipedia.org/wiki/Diabetes - cite_ref-23 Nathan DM, Cleary PA, Backlund JY, *et al.* (December 2005)."Intensive diabetes treatment and cardiovascular disease in patients with type 1 diabetes".*The New England Journal of Medicine* **353** (25): 2643–53.doi:10.1056/NEJMoa052187.PMC 2637991.PMID 16371630.

http://en.wikipedia.org/wiki/Diabetes - cite_ref-24 "The effect of intensive diabetes therapy on the development and progression of neuropathy. The Diabetes Control and Complications Trial Research Group". *Annals of Internal Medicine* **122** (8): 561–8. April 1995. doi:10.1059/0003-4819-122-8-199504150-00001 (inactive 2009-10-31). PMID 7887548.

[a][b] National Institute for Health and Clinical Excellence. *Clinical guideline 66: Type 2 diabetes*. London, 2008.

http://en.wikipedia.org/wiki/Diabetes - cite_ref-26 Adler AI, Stratton IM, Neil HA, *et al.* (August 2000). "Association of systolic blood pressure with macrovascular and microvascular complications of type 2 diabetes (UKPDS 36): prospective observational study". *BMJ* **321**(7258): 412–9.doi:10.1136/bmj.321.7258.412.PMC 27455. PMID 10938049.

a b c Ripsin, CM; Kang, H, Urban, RJ (2009-01-01). "Management of blood glucose in type 2 diabetes mellitus".*American family physician* **79** (1): 29–36. PMID 19145963.

http://en.wikipedia.org/wiki/Diabetes - cite_ref-28 Pignone M, Alberts MJ, Colwell JA, *et al.* (June 2010). "Aspirin for primary prevention of cardiovascular events in people with diabetes: a position statement of the American Diabetes Association, a scientific statement of the American Heart Association, and an expert consensus document of the American College of Cardiology Foundation". *Diabetes Care* **33**(6): 1395–402. doi:10.2337/dc10-0555. PMC 2875463.PMID 20508233.

http://en.wikipedia.org/wiki/Diabetes - cite_ref-29 CDC.gov

http://en.wikipedia.org/wiki/Diabetes - cite_ref-30 "CDC's Diabetes Program-News and Information-Press

Releases-October 26, 2000". Retrieved 2008-06-23.

http://en.wikipedia.org/wiki/Diabetes - cite_ref-31 Narayan KM, Boyle JP, Thompson TJ, Sorensen SW, Williamson DF (October 2003). "Lifetime risk for diabetes mellitus in the United States". *JAMA* **290**(14): 1884–90.doi:10.1001/jama.290.14.1884.PMID 14532317.

http://en.wikipedia.org/wiki/Diabetes - cite_ref-AA2005-Stats_32-0 American Diabetes Association (2005). "Total Prevalence of Diabetes & Pre-diabetes". Archived from the original on 2006-02-08. Retrieved 2006-03-17.

http://en.wikipedia.org/wiki/Diabetes - cite_ref-dlife_33-0 "Seniors and Diabetes".*Elderly And Diabetes-Diabetes and Seniors*. LifeMed Media. 2006. Retrieved 2007-05-14.

http://en.wikipedia.org/wiki/Diabetes - cite_ref-health_34-0 Harris MI, Flegal KM, Cowie CC,*et al.* (April 1998). "Prevalence of diabetes, impaired fasting glucose, and impaired glucose tolerance in U.S. adults. The Third National Health and Nutrition Examination Survey, 1988–1994".*Diabetes Care* **21** (4): 518–24.doi:10.2337/diacare.21.4.518.PMID 9571335.

http://en.wikipedia.org/wiki/Diabetes - cite_ref-35 Australian Institute for Health and Welfare. "Diabetes, an overview". Archived from the original on 2008-06-17. Retrieved 2008-06-23.

[a] [b] Oxford English Dictionary.*diabetes*. Retrieved 2011-06-10.

[a] [b] Harper, Douglas (2001–2010). "Online Etymology Dictionary. *diabetes.*". Retrieved 2011-06-10

[a] [b] [c] [d] [e] [f] Dallas, John (2011)."Royal College of Physicians of Edinburgh. Diabetes, Doctors and Dogs: An exhibition on Diabetes and Endocrinology by the College Library for the 43rd St. Andrew's Day Festival Symposium"

[a] [b] [c] [d] Oxford English Dictionary.*mellite*. Retrieved 2011-06-10.

[a] [b] [c] [d] "MyEtimology.*mellitus.*". Retrieved 2011-06-10

http://en.wikipedia.org/wiki/Diabetes - cite_ref-OED_-ite_41-0 Oxford English Dictionary. *-ite*. Retrieved 2011-06-10.

[a] [b] Dwivedi, Girish & Dwivedi, Shridhar (2007). *History of Medicine: Sushruta – the Clinician – Teacher par Excellence*.National Informatics Centre (Government of India).

http://en.wikipedia.org/wiki/Diabetes - cite_ref-43 Dobson, M. (1776). "Nature of the urine in diabetes". *Medical Observations and Inquiries* **5**: 298–310.

http://en.wikipedia.org/wiki/Diabetes - cite_ref-44 Medvei, Victor Cornelius (1993).*The history of clinical endocrinology*. Carnforth, Lancs., U.K: Parthenon Pub. Group. pp. 23–34. ISBN 1-85070-427-9.

http://en.wikipedia.org/wiki/Diabetes - cite_ref-45 Nabipour, I. (2003). "Clinical Endocrinology in the Islamic Civilization in Iran". *International Journal of Endocrinology and Metabolism* **1**: 43–45 [44–5].

ᵃ ᵇ Patlak M (December 2002)."New weapons to combat an ancient disease: treating diabetes". *The FASEB Journal* **16** (14): 1853. PMID 12468446.

http://en.wikipedia.org/wiki/Diabetes - cite_ref-47 Von Mehring J, Minkowski O. (1890). "Diabetes mellitus nach pankreasexstirpation". *Arch Exp Pathol Pharmakol* **26** (5–6): 371–387. doi:10.1007/BF01831214.

http://en.wikipedia.org/wiki/Diabetes - cite_ref-CanadMedAssocJ1922-Banting_48-0 Banting FG, Best CH, Collip JB, Campbell WR, Fletcher AA (November 1991). "Pancreatic extracts in the treatment of diabetes mellitus: preliminary report. 1922". *CMAJ* **145** (10): 1281–6. PMC 1335942.PMID 1933711.

http://en.wikipedia.org/wiki/Diabetes - cite_ref-Lancet1936-Himsworth_49-0 Himsworth (1936). "*Diabetes mellitus: its differentiation into insulin-sensitive and insulin-insensitive types*". Lancet *i (5864): 127–30. doi:10.1016/S0140-6736(01)36134-2*.

http://en.wikipedia.org/wiki/Diabetes - cite_ref-50 Department of Health (Malta), 1897–1972:Annual Reports.

http://en.wikipedia.org/wiki/Diabetes - cite_ref-51 Yalow RS, Berson SA (July 1960). "Immunoassay of endogenous plasma insulin in man". *The Journal of Clinical Investigation* **39** (7): 1157–75.doi:10.1172/JCI104130.PMC 441860.PMID 13846364.

http://en.wikipedia.org/wiki/Diabetes - cite_ref-52 The Diabetes Control And Complications Trial Research Group (September 1993). "The effect of intensive treatment of diabetes on the development and progression of long-term complications in insulin-dependent diabetes mellitus. The Diabetes Control and Complications Trial Research Group". *The New England Journal of Medicine* **329** (14): 977–86.doi:10.1056/NEJM199309303291401. PMID 8366922.

http://en.wikipedia.org/wiki/Diabetes - cite_ref-53 Theodore H. Tulchinsky, Elena A. Varavikova (2008). *The New Public Health, Second Edition.* New York: Academic Press. p. 200. ISBN 0-12-370890-7.

http://en.wikipedia.org/wiki/Diabetes - cite_ref-54 Piwernetz K, Home PD, Snorgaard O, Antsiferov M, Staehr-Johansen K, Krans M (May 1993). "Monitoring the targets of the St Vincent Declaration and the implementation of quality management in diabetes care: the DIABCARE initiative. The DIABCARE Monitoring Group of the St Vincent Declaration Steering Committee". *Diabetic Medicine* **10** (4): 371–7.doi:10.1111/j.1464-

5491.1993.tb00083.x.PMID 8508624.

http://en.wikipedia.org/wiki/Diabetes - cite_ref-EO005-Dubois.26Bankauskaite_55-0 Dubois, HFW and Bankauskaite, V (2005). "Type 2 diabetes programmes in Europe" (PDF). *Euro Observer* 7 (2): 5–6.

http://en.wikipedia.org/wiki/Diabetes - cite_ref-pmid17563611_56-0 Stewart WF, Ricci JA, Chee E, Hirsch AG, Brandenburg NA (June 2007). "Lost productive time and costs due to diabetes and diabetic neuropathic pain in the US workforce". *J. Occup. Environ. Med.* **49** (6): 672–9. doi:10.1097/JOM.0b013e318065b83a. PMID 17563611.

[a][b] "Diabetes mellitus". *Merck Veterinary Manual, 9th edition (online version).* 2005. Retrieved 2011-10-23.

From Wikipedia, the free encyclopedia
http://en.wikipedia.org/wiki/Diabetes

Three: Symptoms and signs

The main symptoms that you will experience when suffering from burning mouth syndrome are:

Difficulty in sleeping (insomnia). The pain in your mouth may make it hard for you to sleep. And even if you do sleep, when you move while sleeping, the pain may wake you up. This can result in insomnia and adversely affect your health.

Depression. Burning mouth syndrome may take a time of six months to five years to cure. If you are suffering from it, you may start getting depressed because of the length of this condition. A good solution is to indulge yourself in activities of your interest and try not to concentrate on the pain or think about it while it lasts. If you are unable to overcome depression, you may consult a psychiatrist who may then help you get over it.

Problems in eating. Burning mouth syndrome can affect your lips, tongue, gums, roof of the mouth and even the throat; it can get very difficult for you to eat. Taking fluids may be easy but eating solid food may increase the pain. Also, you have to carefully regulate your diet while you are suffering from burning mouth syndrome. For example, while suffering from this condition, you should avoid spicy foods. You should also avoid such fluids which are acidic, such as soft drinks.

Decreased socializing. You may find it hard even to speak at times when the pain is severe. This can force you to stay silent and make you socialize with less and less people so that you may not have to speak. This decreased socializing may also make you get alone and depressed. It may also affect your relationships.

Irritability. If you are a person who is constantly suffering from a paining mouth, there is a huge chance that you will be easily irritated. Many people tend to get cranky when suffering from burning mouth syndrome.

Problems in relationships. This condition can cast bad affect on your relationship if you are not careful. If you let yourself be depressed and be pushed into less socializing by this condition, this may make you a loner and a person who is never happy and always cranky. Other people who love you may get hurt at this attitude and be distanced from you.

Severe pain. The pain may get severe and mild at different times. When severe, it may be sharp and persistent like a tooth-ache pain. It may start in the morning and get severe as the day goes on. In the afternoon, it may become most severe and as the night approaches, it may get less sharp. Pain caused by burning mouth syndrome often affects the tongue and the lips.

Supertasters. This is a common symptom among people who suffer from burning mouth syndrome. If you are suffering from the condition, you may feel that your sense of taste is more enhanced. This happens because the density of your taste buds increases. This makes your tongue more capable to detect a taste than normal is. But this symptom can cause a lot of discomfort. For example, you may feel a food to be very spicy when it's mildly spicy to others.

Four: Meeting the doctor for BMS

Preparing for your appointment with the doctor:

Immediately when the pain starts in your mouth, you will most probably go to see your doctor. Since determining the cause of burning mouth syndrome is a tricky task, your doctor may send you to a specialist for a check-up. The specialist may then diagnose the condition.

You will need to see a number of specialists to properly treat your condition. These include a dermatologist, the skin doctor, a dentist, to diagnose if there's any tooth-related underlying disease, a psychiatrist, to help you cope up with the depression and anxiety that this condition results in and an otolaryngologist, a doctor who specializes in ear, nose and throat, ear and nose problems. Your BMS may be a result of any of a number of diseases. So that's why you may have to visit a number of specialists so that each of them can diagnose you and see if you are suffering from the disease they specialize in. For example, the dentist will check thoroughly to see if you are suffering from dental infection. If you have a fungal, bacterial, or viral infection in your mouth, he will be able to find it out and tell you that it has caused BMS in your case.

Appointments with doctor are very brief and you get a very limited time to ask him anything or to tell him about your problems. So it's always a good idea that you should go to the doctor after planning what you will say and making proper preparations. Here are some tips that may be helpful in letting you use your time with the doctor constructively and making the most of it:

You should know if there are any things you should take care of before the appointment. For example, you must know the names of any medications that you have tried on your own before going to the doctor.

You will have a limited time with the doctor and you may not be able to tell him the symptoms that you are experiencing. Write your symptoms down and as soon as he asks you about them, show him your list. This will make sure that you won't miss any symptoms.

Write down on a page the details of your medical history. The doctor may want to know about it so as to diagnose a possible underlying cause of burning mouth syndrome because it can be a result of different other diseases. So if you had any allergies, infections or medical problems in the past, you should write them down before the appointment and during the appointment, tell the doctor about them.

Write down any important questions that you need to ask the doctor. In the limited time of the appointment, you may miss some of them. Its better that you jot them down before-hand. Some of the important questions that usually should be asked are:

What is the possible cause of your condition? Ask your doctor if it's some other disease, some sort of infection or a dietary imbalance. Often, burning mouth syndrome is an outcome of another underlying disease. So if you have a recent medical history of some sort of infection or a dental operation, you should tell your doctor and then ask him whether it could be the cause of your condition.

Are there any tests that you need to go through? If yes, what are those tests and who will be the right person to carry them out? Also, you may ask the doctor about the probable costs of those tests. This will help you calculate your estimated expenses.

Is the pain in your mouth temporary or will it last for a long time? If your pain is going to be there for a long time, this will help you be mentally prepared for it. You may also start seeing a psychiatrist so that he may help you cope with the prolonged pain.

When your doctor suggests you a medication, do ask

him if there are any alternate medications that can be used in its place. If there are any, ask him why they should or should not be preferred.

Should you see a specialist? For example, if the underlying cause of your burning mouth syndrome is an infection in your teeth, you may be required to meet a dentist. So you should ask your doctor if there's a need to meet any other specialists for your treatment.

Ask your doctor if he has any brochures that you may take home which may be helpful in coping with your condition. For instance, if you are required to take a specific diet while the burning mouth syndrome lasts, your doctor may have a chart of a suitable diet. You should ask him about it and if he has it, request him to give you one.

During the appointment, your doctor may also ask you a number of questions. You should go prepared for them too. Your doctor may ask a question which is important in the diagnosis and if you are not prepared for it, you may not answer it correctly. This can lead to a difficulty in making the right diagnosis. For example, if your burning mouth syndrome is an outcome of some diet imbalance and if your doctor asks you what did you eat a week ago and you are unable to recall, this can result in faulty diagnosis. Given below are a set of questions that you should be mentally prepared for when you go to the doctor:

When did your symptoms first start? Did you change your diet immediately before them? Or did you suffer from any other health problems after which the symptoms began?

Did you make any important change in your life that led to these symptoms? For instance, did you start consuming more alcohol just before the symptoms of BMS appeared? Or did you undergo some situation of shock and trauma? You should be able to answer all these questions since each of them can be a probable cause of BMS and so your doctor must know about them so as to diagnose you correctly.

How severe have your symptoms been? And is their intensity constant or do they become mild some times and severe at others? If they are periodic, are there any specific times when they become severe, for example in the morning or at nights?

Is there anything that improves your symptoms? Any specific kind of food or medication or some other habit?

Is there anything that makes your symptoms worse? It can be some medication, some daily activity, anything at all.

Five: Tests and diagnosis of BMS

There are no specific tests that clearly tell that you have burning mouth syndrome. Your doctor will ask you to undergo a number of tests only so that he can be sure that you are not suffering from any other disease with similar symptoms. When he has sufficiently ruled out other possibilities, he will then diagnose the burning mouth syndrome.

Your doctor will also ask you to tell him your medical history. He will ask you about any medical or health issues that you had in the past and that how did you treat them. He will also ask you if you have recently experienced a situation which caused depression, anxiety or trauma. You may also be asked about your oral hygiene habits. If a dentist has operated on your mouth in the recent past, you should tell the doctor about it too. This is important because in some cases, a fungal infection due to a poor dental operation can be the cause of BMS.

Normally, the tests that your doctor will ask you to undergo during the diagnosis of burning mouth syndrome are:

Blood tests:

Through the blood tests, the doctor will make sure that your blood glucose level, complete blood count, immune functioning and other nutritional elements are at a normal level. If they are at an abnormal level, this will give the doctor a clue about the cause of your condition. If the levels are normal, the doctor will know that nothing in your blood has caused the condition.

Imaging:

You may be asked by your doctor to get a magnetic-resonance-imaging (MRI) or a computed tomography (CT) scan. This will help the doctor determine if you have any other health problems.

Oral check-up:

You may be asked to provide samples from your mouth. These samples will then be checked with different chemicals to see if you have any bacterial, fungal or viral infections. During the oral check-up, the doctor will also see if your mouth is sensitive to any artificial material, like dentures, if you are using them. In some cases, your mouth may be sensitive to dentures and mouth cells may show some sort of reaction. It can be the cause of BMS. During the oral check-up, the doctor will try to see if such a reaction exists within your mouth.

Saliva measurement:

Dry mouth is a condition in which the glands in your mouth producing saliva don't produce normal amounts. It is more common in elderly people. This can lead to a feeling of a dry mouth. If you are suffering from this condition, you may also feel a metallic taste on your tongue when eating food. In some cases, this may even be the cause of burning mouth syndrome. In other cases, it is a symptom of burning mouth syndrome. The saliva measurements help the doctor determine whether or not your saliva flow is abnormal. If it is less than normal, he will prescribe you the appropriate medication that boasts saliva production.

Allergy tests:

Your doctor may ask you to undergo a number of allergy tests. These tests will check whether or not you are allergic to specific foods or substances. In case you had a dental operation in the past and have an artificial part in your tooth, these tests will check if your mouth is allergic to it. Allergy tests may take a long time because you can be allergic to a lot of things and you may not even know about it. So, through allergy tests, the doctor has to find it out through hit-and-trial method. In such a method, the doctor suggests you a medicine and if it doesn't make any improvements to your symptoms, he asks you to stop using it and suggests another. And so on until he finds the right medicine that can improve your symptoms.

Psychological questionnaires:

Burning mouth syndrome can be a long-term disease and it can take from six months up to five years to cure. Due to this, you may start suffering from depression and anxiety and stop socializing with other people. This condition may also affect your relationships with your close ones. Psychological diagnosis is an important way of checking whether or not this condition is having any adverse psychological effects on you. You may be asked to fill out a questionnaire that asks different questions regarding your mental state. The answers to these questions may reveal to a psychiatrist if you are suffering from any psychological problems.

Gastric reflux tests:

Gastric reflux is a condition in which the acid produced by the stomach rises through the food-pipe that carries food from mouth to the stomach. This causes a burning sensation in the chest. This can often cause burning mouth syndrome. Gastric reflux tests check if you are suffering from this condition.

Six: Treatment

There is no definite treatment for burning mouth syndrome. The treatment is actually aimed at curing the causes of this condition.   In different people, different factors may cause burning mouth syndrome. And it may show different signs and symptoms. Any of the many diseases mentioned above may by the underlying cause of your condition. So it is very important to find that cause and diagnose it correctly because the treatment is focused to eliminating that cause and treating it.

There are two types of burning mouth syndrome, primary and secondary. In the primary type, the doctor is unable to find the cause of your condition. In secondary type, some other disease is the cause of your condition. So if you are suffering from primary condition, it can become very difficult for the doctor to suggest any medications for you. Because he doesn't even know what is causing it. In such a case, it's a hit-and-trial method. The doctor suggests a medication and if it doesn't work, he suggests another. And so on, until some medication starts to improve your condition.

The treatment options for burning mouth syndrome may include the following medications:

Oral thrush medications. These medications treat any fungal infections that may be affecting your teeth, e.g., nystatin.

Saliva replacement products. These help you get over the feeling of dry mouth. A number of other medications may also help in treating dry mouth. These include low dosages of clonazepam (Klonopin), chlordiazepoxide (Librium), tricyclic antidepressants and gabapentin (Neurontin).

Vitamin B complex. These are done so that if your burning mouth syndrome is a result of deficiency in nutrients, they may be replaced through these vitamins.

Antidepressants. As in some cases, burning mouth syndrome can be a result of severe depression, anxiety and trauma, these antidepressant medications help you get over such depression.

Capsaicin. A medicine that helps in relieving pain and it is derived from chili peppers.

Oral mouthwashes. These clean the mouth and prevent any chances of fungal or viral infections.

Anticonvulsant medication, e.g., clonazepam

(Klonopin). These drugs are helpful in treating the pain symptoms of burning mouth syndrome.

Oral supplements. These are medicines which help in restoring the nutritional deficiencies in your body. An example is the tablets containing iron or calcium.

Other medications that your doctor may advise you to use when treating burning mouth syndrome are:

A 10mg dose of tricyclic antidepressants at bedtime. After every four to seven days, increase the dose by 10 mg. Keep on increasing the dose until the feeling of burning in mouth is relieved or some side-effects start to appear.

0.25 mg of Clonazepam at bedtime. After every four to seven days, increase the dose by 0.25 mg. Keep on increasing the dose until the feeling of burning is relieved or some side-effects occur. As you increase dose amounts, you should start taking them three divided doses daily.

5 mg of Chlordiazepoxide at bedtime. After every four to seven days, increase the dose by 5 mg. Keep on increasing the dose until the feeling of burning is relieved or some side-effects occur. As dosages increases, you should take the medicine in three equally divided doses daily.

100 mg of Gabapentin at bedtime. After every four to seven days, increase the dose by 100 mg. Keep on increasing the dose until the feeling of burning is relieved or some side-effects occur. As dosages increases, you should take the

medicine in three equally divided doses daily.

Seven: Lifestyle Changes

Burning mouth syndrome is a long-term disease. It may take months or even years to completely go away, depending upon the severity and the causes. While it lasts, you must change your lifestyle so that you may be able to cope best with your condition. Here are some tips through which you can ensure that this condition has minimum adverse affects on your life:

Try to drink more fluids: specifically, water. This will help you reduce the feeling of dry mouth. But you should be careful not to take acidic fluids or foods because they may worsen your condition.

You may change different habits to see if they help in reducing the pain in your mouth. For example, you may change toothpaste brands to see which one suits your teeth and mouth most. Ideally, a brand to which your teeth or mouth shows no sensitivity and which results in no side-effects is the best brand for you.

You should try not to eat spicy and hot foods. They may worsen the pain in your mouth and throat.

Avoid products that contain tobacco such as cigarettes. Such products can complicate your condition and prolong it.

Try not to take acidic food or fluids and liquids such as soft drinks, tomato juice, or coffee.

Avoid products with cinnamon or mint.

Try to take steps to reduce your anxiety. Anxiety can cause burning mouth syndrome and it can also prolong the treatment if you take no steps to reduce it. There are a number of ways to reduce your anxiety levels. For example, take up yoga or visit a psychiatrist who may help you reduce stress.

Engage in activities which make you feel good. This will help you ignore the pain and cope with it. For example, if you like watching movies, tune into your favorite movie when your pain gets severe. This may help you overcome it. Also, if you are feeling depressed or anxious because of your condition, indulge in something you enjoy doing. You may, for instance, go meet some really good friend or read an interesting novel.

Socialize. Depression and anxiety are some of the most prominent symptoms of burning mouth syndrome. They can push you into loneliness as you start avoiding people when you are depressed. This can ruin your social life and also affect your relationships. So you must do a conscious effort to counter this. You should try to socialize and be friends with others, try to discuss different things and not push yourself into a corner because of your condition.

Try not to use mouthwashes which contain alcohol.

Avoid toothpastes which contain sodium lauryl sulfate.

Chew sugarless gum. This will help you in easing the pain and in coping with dry mouth.

If you are suffering from burning mouth syndrome, the pain you experience in your mouth will be mild in the morning when you wake up. Then as the day goes on, it will probably become worse. By the afternoon, the pain will become most severe. And then, as night approaches, it will lessen again. So you should brace yourself for the pain in the afternoon and take up some relaxing activity so that at that particular time when the pain is most severe, you can somehow cope with it.

Sometimes, the pain in your mouth may disturb your sleep. It may start at night so you may feel unable to sleep. This can lead to insomnia and cause mood swings and crankiness. You should be prepared about it and know how to tackle it if it happens. For instance, you may put on a soft, melodious music when you want to go to sleep. It may help you overcome the pain and doze off to sleep more easily.

Glossary of Medical Terms

Abnormal: Not normal. Deviating from the usual position, condition, structure or behavior. An abnormal growth could indicate a premalignant or malignant condition. In other words, an abnormal growth could indicate cancer

Acquired: An acquired condition is one that isn't present at birth. In other words, it is a condition that is not inherited.

Acute: A condition with an abrupt onset. A brain aneurism is said to be acute if it comes on suddenly. An acute condition could also describe an illness of short duration that rapidly progresses and requires urgent care.

Airway: The trachea. A method of preventing sensation, used to eliminate pain. The loss or prevention of pain, as caused by anesthesia.

Aneurysm or Aneurism: An abnormal blood-filled swelling of an artery or vein, resulting from a localized weakness in the wall of the vessel.

Angiography: A medical imaging technique in which an X-ray image is taken to visualize the inside of blood vessels and organs of the body, with particular interest in the arteries, veins and the heart chambers.

Artery: An efferent blood vessel from the heart, conveying blood away from the heart regardless of oxygenation status.

Autopsy: A dissection performed on a cadaver to find possible cause(s) of death. An after-the-fact examination, especially of the causes of a failure.

Berry aneurysm: An aneurism that looks like a berry. It usually happens where a cerebral artery leaves the circular artery at the base of the brain.

Blood pressure: The pressure exerted by the blood against the walls of the arteries and veins; it varies during the heartbeat cycle, and according to a person's age, health and physical condition. The great majority of people who have serious conditions from high blood pressure suffer debilitating illness.

Brain: The control center of the central nervous system of an animal located in the skull which is responsible for perception, cognition, attention, memory, emotion, and action.

Brain aneurysm: See berry aneurysm.

Brain swelling: See: Cerebral edema.

Breathing: The act of respiration; a single instance of this.

Calcium: A mineral stored in the bones. Calcium is added to bones by osteoblasts and is removed osteoclasts. This mineral s essential for healthy bones and regulates muscle contraction, heart action, nervous system maintenance, and normal blood clotting. Food sources of calcium include dairy foods, some leafy green vegetables such as broccoli and collards, canned salmon, clams, oysters, calcium-fortified foods, and tofu.

Calcium channel blocker: A drug that blocks calcium from entering the heart and artery muscle, preventing narrowing of the arteries.

Cardiovascular: Relating to the circulatory system, that is the heart and blood vessels.

Catheter: small tube inserted into a body cavity to remove fluid, create an opening, distend a passageway or administer a drug

Cell: The basic unit of a living organism, surrounded by a cell membrane.

Cerebral: Of, or relating to the brain or cerebral cortex of the brain.

Cerebral aneurysm: See: Berry aneurysm.

Cholesterol: A sterollipid synthesized by the liver and transported in the bloodstream to the membranes of all animal cells; it plays a central role in many biochemical processes and, as a lipoprotein that coats the walls of blood vessels, is associated with cardiovascular disease.

Circle of Willis: An arterial circle at the base of the brain. Circulation: The movement of the blood in the blood-vascular system, by which it is brought into close relations with almost every living elementary constituent.

Cocaine: A stimulant narcotic in the form of a white powder that users generally self-administer by insufflation through the nose. Any derivative of cocaine. Extracted from the leaves of the coca scrub (Erythroxylon coca) indigenous to the Andean highlands of South America.

Coma: A state of sleep from which one may not wake up, usually induced by some form of trauma.

Compression (medicine): Pressing together. As in a compression fracture, nerve compression , or spinal cord compression.

Compression (embryology): To shorten in time.

Connective tissue: type of tissue found in animals whose main function is binding other tissue systems (such as muscle to skin) or organs and consists of the following three elements: cells, fibers and a ground substance (or extracellular matrix).

Contrast: Any substance, such as barium sulfate, used in radiography to increase the visibility of internal structures

CT scan: Computerized tomography scan. Pictures of the body created by a computer where multiple X-ray images are turned into pictures on a screen.

Cysts: A pouch or sac without opening, usually membranous and containing morbid matter, which develops in one of the natural cavities or in the substance of an organ.

Dizziness: he state of being dizzy; the sensation of instability.

Doppler ultrasound: A type of ultrasound that detects and measures blood flow.

Ehlers-Danlos syndrome: A heritable disorder of connective tissue with easy bruising, joint hypermobility (loose joints), skin laxity, and weakness of tissues.

Emergency department: The department of a hospital that

treats emergencies.

Extended family: a family consisting of parents and children, along with either grandparents, grandchildren, aunts or uncles etc.

Extremity: the most extreme or furthest point of something.

1. An extreme measure.

2. A hand or foot.

Genetic: (genetics) relating to genetics or genes. Caused by genes.

Groin: The long narrow depression of the human body that separates the trunk from the legs.

Headache: A pain or ache in the head.

Hemorrhage: A heavy release of blood within or from the body.

High blood pressure: Hypertension: a repeatedly elevated blood pressure exceeding 140 over 90 mmHg -- a systolic pressure above 140 with a diastolic pressure above 90.

Inheritance: The hereditary passing of biological attributes from ancestors to their offspring.

Interventional: Intervening, interfering or interceding with the intent of modifying the outcome. For example, an interventional radiologist.

Intracranial: f or pertaining to the brain or inside of the head. Within the cranium.

Kidney: an organ in the body that produces urine.

Lifetime risk: The risk of developing a particular disease or dying from that disease during your lifetime.

Long-term memory: Permanent storage, management, and retrieval of information for later use.

Lumbar: Related to the lower back or loin.

Lumbar puncture: A diagnostic and at times therapeutic procedure performed to collect a sample of cerebrospinal fluid for biochemical, microbiological, and cytological analysis, or rarely to relieve increased intracranial pressure.

Marfan syndrome: A genetic disorder of the connective tissue that causes defects in the heart valves and aorta. Characterized by abnormalities of the eyes, skeleton, and cardiovascular system.

Memory: 1. The ability to recover information about past events or knowledge. 2. The process of recovering information about past events or knowledge. 3. Cognitive reconstruction. The brain engages in a remarkable reshuffling process in an attempt to extract what is general and what is particular about each passing moment.

Migraine: Usually, periodic attacks of headaches on one or both sides of the head. These may be accompanied by nausea, vomiting, increased sensitivity of the eyes to light (photophobia), increased sensitivity to sound (phonophobia), dizziness, blurred vision, cognitive disturbances, and other symptoms. Some migraines do not include headache, and migraines may or may not be preceded by an aura.

MRI: Abbreviation and nickname for magnetic resonance imaging. For more information, see: Magnetic Resonance Imaging; Paul C. Lauterbur ; Peter Mansfield .

Nausea: Nausea, is the urge to vomit. It can be brought by many causes including, systemic illnesses, such as influenza, medications, pain, and inner ear disease. When nausea and/or vomiting are persistent, or when they are accompanied by other severe symptoms such as abdominal pain, jaundice , fever, or bleeding, a physician should be consulted.

Neck: The part of the body joining the head to the shoulders. Also, any narrow or constricted part of a bone or organ that joins its parts as, for example, the neck of the femur bone.

Nerve: A bundle of fibers that uses chemical and electrical signals to transmit sensory and motor information from one body part to another. See: Nervous system.

Nerve cell: See: Neuron.

Neurofibromatosis: A genetic disorder of the nervous system that primarily affects the development and growth of neural (nerve) cell tissues, causes tumors to grow on nerves, and may produce other abnormalities.

Neurological: Having to do with the nerves or the nervous system.

Neurology: The medical specialty concerned with the diagnosis and treatment of disorders of the nervous system -- the brain, the spinal cord, and the nerves.

Neuroradiology: The field within radiology that specializes in the use of radioactive substances, x-rays and scanning devices for the diagnosis and treatment of diseases of the nervous system. Neuroradiology involves the clinical imaging, therapy, and basic science of the central and peripheral nervous system , including but not limited to the brain, spine , head and neck , interventional procedures, techniques in imaging and intervention , and related educational, socioeconomic, and medicolegal issues.

Neurosurgeon: A physician trained in surgery of the nervous system and who specializes in surgery on the brain and other parts of the nervous system. Sometimes called a "brain surgeon."

NIH: The National Institutes of Health. The NIH is an important U.S. health agency. It is devoted to medical research. Administratively under the Department of Health and Human Services (HHS), the NIH consists of 20-some separate Institutes and Centers. NIH's program activities are represented by these Institutes and Centers.

Onset: In medicine, the first appearance of the signs or symptoms of an illness as, for example, the onset of rheumatoid arthritis. There is always an onset to a disease but never to the return to good health. The default setting is good health.

Outpatient: A patient who is not an inpatient (not hospitalized) but instead is cared for elsewhere -- as in a doctor's office, clinic, or day surgery center. The term outpatient dates back at least to 1715. Outpatient care today is also called ambulatory care.

Pain: An unpleasant sensation that can range from mild,

localized discomfort to agony. Pain has both physical and emotional components. The physical part of pain results from nerve stimulation. Pain may be contained to a discrete area, as in an injury, or it can be more diffuse, as in disorders like fibromyalgia. Pain is mediated by specific nerve fibers that carry the pain impulses to the brain where their conscious appreciation may be modified by many factors.

Pharmacy: A location where prescription drugs are sold. A pharmacy is, by law, constantly supervised by a licensed pharmacist.

Polycystic kidney disease: One of the genetic disorders characterized by the development of innumerable cysts in the kidneys. These cysts are filled with fluid, and replace much of the mass of the kidneys. This reduces kidney function, leading to kidney failure.

Pupil: The opening of the iris. The pupil may appear to open (dilate) and close (constrict) but it is really the iris that is the prime mover; the pupil is merely the absence of iris. The pupil determines how much light is let into the eye. Both pupils are usually of equal size. If they are not, that is termed anisocoria (from "a-", not + "iso", equal + "kore", pupil = not equal pupils).

Radiologic: Having to do with radiology.

Radiologist: A physician specialized in radiology, the branch of medicine that uses ionizing and nonionizing radiation for the diagnosis and treatment of disease.

Residual: Something left behind. With residual disease, the disease has not been eradicated.

Risk factor: Something that increases a person's chances of developing a disease.

Rupture: A break or tear in any organ (such as the spleen) or soft tissue (such as the achilles tendon). Rupture of the appendix is more likely among uninsured and minority children when they develop appendicitis.

Saccular: From the Latin "sacculus" meaning a small pouch. As for example the alveolar saccules (little air pouches) within the lungs.

Saccular aneurysm: An aneurysm that resembles a small sack. A berry aneurysm is typically saccular. An aneurysm is a localized widening (dilatation) of an artery, vein, or the heart. At the area of an aneurysm, there is typically a bulge and the wall is weakened and may rupture. The word "aneurysm" comes from the Greek "aneurysma" meaning "a widening."

Scan: As a noun, the data or image obtained from the examination of organs or regions of the body by gathering information with a sensing device.

Seizure: Uncontrolled electrical activity in the brain, which may produce a physical convulsion, minor physical signs, thought disturbances, or a combination of symptoms.

Sensitivity: 1. In psychology, the quality of being sensitive. As, for example, sensitivity training, training in small groups to develop a sensitive awareness and understanding of oneself and of ones relationships with others. 2. In disease epidemiology, the ability of a system to detect epidemics and other changes in disease occurrence. 3. In screening for a disease, the proportion of persons with the disease who are correctly identified by a screening test. 4. In the definition of a disease, the proportion of persons with the disease who are correctly identified by defined criteria.

Skull: The skull is a collection of bones which encase the brain and give form to the head and face. The bones of the skull include the following: the frontal, parietal, occipital, temporal, sphenoid, ethmoid, zygomatic, maxilla, nasal, vomer, palatine, inferior concha, and mandible.

Spasm: A brief, automatic jerking movement. A muscle spasm can be quite painful, with the muscle clenching tightly. A spasm of the coronary artery can cause angina. Spasms in various types of tissue may be caused by stress, medication, over-exercise, or other factors.

Spinal cord: The major column of nerve tissue that is connected to the brain and lies within the vertebral canal and from which the spinal nerves emerge. Thirty-one pairs of spinal nerves originate in the spinal cord: 8 cervical, 12 thoracic , 5 lumbar, 5 sacral, and 1 coccygeal. The spinal cord and the brain constitute the central nervous system (CNS). The spinal cord consists of nerve fibers that transmit impulses to and from the brain. Like the brain, the spinal cord is covered by three connective-tissue envelopes called the meninges . The space between the outer and middle envelopes is filled with cerebrospinal fluid (CSF), a clear colorless fluid that cushions the spinal cord against jarring shock. Also known simply as the cord.

Spinal tap: Also known as a lumbar puncture or "LP", a spinal tap is a procedure whereby spinal fluid is removed from the spinal canal for the purpose of diagnostic testing. It is particularly helpful in the diagnosis of inflammatory diseases of the central nervous system, especially infections, such as meningitis. It can also provide clues to the diagnosis of stroke, spinal cord tumor and cancer in the central nervous system.

Stress: Forces from the outside world impinging on the

individual. Stress is a normal part of life that can help us learn and grow. Conversely, stress can cause us significant problems.

Stroke: The sudden death of some brain cells due to a lack of oxygen when the blood flow to the brain is impaired by blockage or rupture of an artery to the brain. A stroke is also called a cerebrovascular accident or, for short, a CVA.

Subarachnoid: Literally, beneath the arachnoid, the middle of three membranes that cover the central nervous system. In practice, subarachnoid usually refers to the space between the arachnoid and the pia mater, the innermost membrane surrounding the central nervous system.

Subarachnoid hemorrhage: Bleeding within the head into the space between two membranes that surround the brain. The bleeding is beneath the arachnoid membrane and just above the pia mater. (The arachnoid is the middle of three membranes around the brain while the pia mater is the innermost one.)

Surgery: The word "surgery" has multiple meanings. It is the branch of medicine concerned with diseases and conditions which require or are amenable to operative procedures. Surgery is the work done by a surgeon. By analogy, the work of an editor wielding his pen as a scalpel is s form of surgery.

A surgery in England (and some other countries) is a physician's or dentist's office.

Swelling of the brain: See: Cerebral edema.

Symptom: Any subjective evidence of disease. Anxiety, lower back pain, and fatigue are all symptoms. They are sensations only the patient can perceive. In contrast, a sign is objective evidence of disease. A bloody nose is a sign. It is evident to the patient, doctor, nurse and other observers.

Syndrome: A set of signs and symptoms that tend to occur together and which reflect the presence of a particular disease or an increased chance of developing a particular disease.

Temple: An area just behind and to the side of the forehead and the eye, above the side of the check bone (the zygomatic arch) and in front of the ear.

Tension: 1) The pressure within a vessel, such as blood pressure: the pressure within the blood vessels. For example, elevated blood pressure is referred to as hypertension. 2) Stress, especially stress that is translated into clenched scalp muscles and bottled-up emotions or anxiety. This is the type of tension blamed for tension headaches.

Therapeutic: Relating to therapeutics, that part of medicine concerned specifically with the treatment of disease. The therapeutic dose of a drug is the amount needed to treat a disease.

Throat: The throat is the anterior (front) portion of the neck beginning at the back of the mouth , consisting anatomically of the pharynx and larynx . The throat contains the trachea and a portion of the esophagus.

Tobacco: A South American herb, formally known as Nicotiana tabacum, whose leaves contain 2-8% nicotine and serve as the source of smoking and smokeless tobacco.

Transcranial: Through the cranium. As, for example, in transcranial magnetic stimulation.

Ultrasound : High-frequency sound waves. Ultrasound waves can be bounced off of tissues using special devices. The echoes are then converted into a picture called a sonogram. Ultrasound imaging, referred to as ultrasonography, allows physicians and patients to get an inside view of soft tissues and body cavities, without using invasive techniques. Ultrasound is often used to examine a fetus during pregnancy There is no convincing evidence for any danger from ultrasound during pregnancy.

Vessel: A tube in the body that carries fluids: blood vessels or lymph vessels.

Visual field: The entire area that can be seen when the eye is directed forward, including that which is seen with peripheral vision.

X-ray: 1. High-energy radiation with waves shorter than those of visible light. X-rays possess the properties of penetrating most substances (to varying extents), of acting on a photographic film or plate (permitting radiography), and of causing a fluorescent screen to give off light (permitting fluoroscopy). In low doses X-rays are used for making images that help to diagnose disease, and in high doses to treat cancer. Formerly called a Roentgen ray. 2. An image obtained by means of X-rays.

Appendix A: Internet Resources / Further Reading

The following Internet resources may be helpful in answering any health or medical questions you may have. The sites were chosen because of their superior content, accuracy, and authority.

Print Publications Online

American Family Physician
<http://www.aafp.org/online/en/home/publications/journals/afp.html>
A full-text, online version of the esteemed journal. Contains excellent review articles on clinical medicine. Many come with patient education information.

Merck Manual of Diagnosis and Therapy, 17th ed.
<http://www.merck.com/mmpe/index.html>

A medical guide for professionals, available online. Contains technical information for a host of diseases along with their corresponding diagnosis and treatment suggestions.

Merck Manual of Geriatrics
<http://www.merck.com/mkgr/mmg/home.jsp>

Similar in format to the Merck Manual of Diagnosis and
Therapy, this guide focuses on disorders and diseases with a
slant towards implications for the elderly.

Merck Manual of Medical Information - 2nd Home Edition
<http://www.merck.com/mmhe/index.html>

A consumers' guide to diseases and their treatments. This is a
complete online version of the text edition, with videos and a
pronunciation guide

Postgraduate Medicine
<http://www.postgradmed.com/>
Professional medical journal with review articles on diseases
and treatments. Although this is directed to the professional,
the journal includes patient notes which are directed toward
the general consumer.

MEDLINE/MedlinePlus
<http://www.nlm.nih.gov/medlineplus/>

Anatomy videos aimed at the general consumer plus
thousands of articles on a variety of health related topics.

PubMed
<http://www.ncbi.nlm.nih.gov/sites/entrez>
PubMed comprises more than 20 million citations for
biomedical literature from MEDLINE, life science journals,
and online books. Citations may include links to full-text
content from PubMed Central and publisher web sites.

News Services
These sources offer reliable information and up to date news

stories about medical research.

Understanding Medical News

Consumer's Guide to Taking Charge of Medical Information
<http://www.health-insight-harvard.org/>

This guide, developed by the Harvard School of Public Health, helps you to decipher "scary" headlines.

Deciphering Medspeak
<http://mlanet.org/resources/medspeak/index.html>

To make informed health decisions, you have probably read a newspaper or magazine article, tuned into a radio or television program, or searched the Internet to find answers to health questions. If so, you have probably encountered "medspeak," the specialized language of health professionals. The Medical Library Association developed "Deciphering Medspeak" to help translate common "medspeak" terms.

HealthNewsReviews
<http://www.healthnewsreview.org/>
HealthNewsReview.org is a website dedicated to:
- Improving the accuracy of news stories about medical treatments, tests, products and procedures.
- Helping consumers evaluate the evidence for and against new ideas in health care.

Interpreting News on Diet and Nutrition
<http://www.hsph.harvard.edu/nutritionsource/nutrition-news/media/>

Confused by all the conflicting stories about what's good to eat and what's not? Sensational headlines don't always tell the whole story. Look at how nutrition news fits into the bigger scientific picture.

Understanding Risk. What Do Those Headlines Really Mean?
<http://www.niapublications.org/tipsheets/pdf/Understanding_Risk-What_Do_Those_Headlines_Really_Mean.pdf>

Tipsheet that discusses the differences among types of clinical research and explains the significance of types of risk in research results. Excellent easy to understand information about risk.

Beyond the Headlines: What Consumers Need To Know About Nutrition News
<http://www.foodinsight.org/>

The International Food Information Council Foundation is dedicated to the mission of effectively communicating science-based information on health, food safety and nutrition for the public good.

Recommended Online News Sources

Aetna InteliHealth Health News
<http://www.intelihealth.com/IH/ihtIH/WSIHW000/333/333.html?k=menux408x333>

Top news headlines for the day. There is a section with commentaries written by Harvard Medical School physicians of several of the day's top news stories.

CNN Health
<http://www.cnn.com/HEALTH/>

Daily updated articles from a variety of news sources with links to related CNN stories and websites.

1st Headlines - Top Health Headlines
<http://www.1stheadlines.com/health.htm>

Top news stories from a variety of sources. Story may be covered by more than one news sources, allowing you to compare stories and fill in information gaps.

Reuters Health eLine
<http://www.reutershealth.com/en/index.html>

Daily medical news for the consumer (free) and for the professional (requires a subscription fee).

News Sources with Daily or Weekly Email Delivery

MedlinePlus Health News
<http://www.nlm.nih.gov/medlineplus/>

Produced by the National Library of Medicine, this site has daily news releases from sources such as United Press International, New York Times Syndicate, and Reuters. Stories can be retrieved for thirty days from publication. Users may sign up for daily email of "Health Headlines" in several different categories.

Medscape
<http://www.medscape.com/>

From WebMD, a website for doctors with a comprehensive

news feature. Go to the website to read the daily news or sign up for any of the forty free newsletters for delivery to your email address. There are newsletters in twenty-five specialties, a weekly multi-specialty edition, health business news, and much more.

NewsWise
<http://feeds.feedburner.com/NewswiseMednews>
Medical news stories. Information from news releases of more than four hundred universities, professional associations, and research institutions. Register and sign up to receive weekly medical news digests via email.

Alternative Medicine Ask Dr. Weil
<http://www.drweil.com/>

The popular doctor discusses alternative healing remedies for many common ailments.

Alternative Medicine Homepage
<http://www.pitt.edu/~cbw/altm.html>
From the Falk Library of the Health Sciences, University of Pittsburgh - a jumpstation for sources of information on unconventional, alternative, complementary, innovative, and integrative therapies.

HerbMed

<http://www.herbmed.org/>

HerbMed is an interactive, electronic herbal database. It provides hyperlinked access to the scientific & medical research articles on the use of herbs for treating medical conditions. This evidence-based information resource is for professionals, researchers, and the general public.

National Center for Complementary and Alternative Medicine
<http://nccam.nih.gov/>

General information about alternative and complementary therapies with links to research studies currently being conducted on alternative therapies for a variety of conditions.

Rosenthal Center for Complementary and Alternative Medicine
<http://www.rosenthal.hs.columbia.edu/>

Links to resources on acupuncture, homeopathy, chiropractic, and herbal medicine and alternative therapies for cancer and women's health. The Center sponsors research on alternative and complementary medical practices.

Clinical Research Trials

Center Watch
<http://www.centerwatch.com/>

Information on over 41,000 clinical trials for twenty disease categories. Profiles of 150 research centers conducting clinical trials and profiles of companies that provide a variety of contract services to the clinical trials industry. Includes industry and government sponsored clinical trials and information on new drug treatments approved by the Food and Drug Administration.

Clinical Trials
<http://www.clinicaltrials.gov/>

Information on current research being conducted on treatments for different diseases. Browse by disease category and sponsor or search the entire site. Learn what clinical trials are all about and how to decide to participate in a trial.

Diseases, Medical Conditions, General Health

Aetna Intelihealth
<http://www.intellihealth.com/IH/ihtIH?t=408>

From the Harvard Medical School, information on diseases and medical conditions, health and fitness, medications, nutrition, childbirth, and other topics.

Healthfinder
<http://www.healthfinder.gov/>

From the U.S. Department of Health and Human Services, a gateway to consumer information on diseases, medical conditions, health promotion, and many other topics.

Mayo Clinic

<http://www.mayoclinic.com/>

From the famed Mayo Clinic, information on diseases and conditions, treatment decisions, drugs and supplements, healthy living, and health assessment tools. Special features include online videos of exercises, diagnostic tests, surgical procedures, and medical conditions, healthy recipes, and self-care information.

National Organization for Rare Diseases

<http://www.rarediseases.org/>

Basic information on rare diseases and disorders. Full-reports are available for a fee.

NOAH (New York Online Access to Health)
<http://www.noah-health.org/>

English and Spanish language information and resources from organizations and governmental agencies. Aging, cancer, asthma, eye diseases, foot and ankle disorders, and pain are just a few of the topics covered.

Health Care Providers

American Board of Medical Specialties (ABMS)
<http://www.abms.org/>

Verify the certification status of any physician in the 24 specialities of the ABMS. Registration is required (free) and user is limited to five searches in a 24 hour period.

AMA Physician Select
<https://extapps.ama-assn.org/doctorfinder/recaptcha.jsp>

Gives credentials of MD's and DO's including medical school, year of graduation, and specialties.

American Hospital Directory
<http://www.ahd.com/>

Profiles of U.S. hospitals. Basic service is free; more detailed information by paid subscription only.

Federation of State Medical Boards
<http://www.fsmb.org/>

Select "Public Services" from the left-hand index, then select "Directory of State Medical Boards" to find links to web sites for the 50 U.S. States, plus the District of Columbia, Guam, and the Northern Mariana Islands. Not all of the states have physician profile or disciplinary action information. There are also links to osteopathic physician sites when available.

Health Pages
<http://www.healthpages.com/>

Information about physicians, dentists, hospitals and clinics, elder care facilities, dietitians and nutritionists.

Joint Commission on the Accreditation of Healthcare Organizations
<http://www.jointcommission.org/>
The Quality Check feature on this site supplies details on individual hospital performance ratings from JCAHO's accreditation reports. View Performance Reports and compare institutions' ratings. Reports cover hospitals, nursing homes, ambulatory care facilities, home care, laboratory services, and long term care facilities.

Nursing Home Compare
<http://www.medicare.gov/NHCompare/Include/DataSection/Questions/SearchCriteriaNEW.asp?version=default&browser=Chrome|6|WinNT&language=English&defaultstatus

=0&pagelist=Home&CookiesEnabledStatus=True>
Provides detailed information about the performance of every Medicare and Medicaid certified nursing home in the country. Searchable by state. Includes a guide to choosing a nursing home and a nursing home checklist to help in making informed choices.

Questions and Answers about Health Insurance: A Consumer Guide

<http://www.ahrq.gov/consumer/insuranceqa/>

Questions and answers on choosing and using a health plan.

Quackery and Health Fraud

Quackwatch
<http://www.quackwatch.com/>

Want information about whether those alternative therapies work? This site has information on health fraud, medical quackery, "new age" medicine and "alternative" and "complementary" medicine.

National Council against Health Fraud
<http://www.ncahf.org/>
Non-profit voluntary health agency focusing on health fraud, misinformation, and quackery as public health oncerns. Read their position papers on acupuncture, homepathy, chiropractic, and other health issues.

Surgery

American College of Surgeons
<http://www.facs.org/>
 Public information section offers guidelines on choosing a qualified surgeon.

Tests and Procedures - MedlinePlus

<http://www.nlm.nih.gov/medlineplus/tutorial.html>
Interactive tutorials on 24 common tests and diagnostic procedures and more than 30 surgeries and treatment procedures.

CPSIA information can be obtained
at www.ICGtesting.com
Printed in the USA
LVOW04s2341130716
496244LV00033B/892/P